T0348627

Ear, Nose, and Throat Emergencies

Editors

LAURA J. BONTEMPO
JAN SHOENBERGER

EMERGENCY MEDICINE CLINICS OF NORTH AMERICA

www.emed.theclinics.com

Consulting Editor
AMAL MATTU

February 2019 • Volume 37 • Number 1

ELSEVIER

1600 John F. Kennedy Boulevard • Suite 1800 • Philadelphia, Pennsylvania, 19103-2899

http://www.theclinics.com

EMERGENCY MEDICINE CLINICS OF NORTH AMERICA Volume 37, Number 1
February 2019 ISSN 0733-8627, ISBN-13: 978-0-323-65453-1

Editor: Colleen Dietzler
Developmental Editor: Casey Potter

Emergency Medicine Clinics of North America (ISSN 0733-8627) is published quarterly by Elsevier Inc., 360 Park Avenue South, New York, NY, 10010-1710. Months of issue are February, May, August, and November. Business and Editorial Offices: 1600 John F. Kennedy Boulevard, Suite 1800, Philadelphia, PA 19103-2899. Customer Service Office: 6277 Sea Harbor Drive, Orlando, FL 32887-4800. Periodicals postage paid at New York, NY, and additional mailing offices. Subscription prices are $100.00 per year (US students), $349.00 per year (US individuals), $679.00 per year (US institutions), $220.00 per year (international students), $462.00 per year (international individuals), $836.00 per year (international institutions), $220.00 per year (Canadian students), $411.00 per year (Canadian individuals), and $836.00 per year (Canadian institutions). International air speed delivery is included in all *Clinics'* subscription prices. All prices are subject to change without notice. POSTMASTER: Send address changes to *Emergency Medicine Clinics of North America*, Elsevier Periodicals Customer Service, 11830 Westline Industrial Drive, St. Louis, MO 63146. Customer Service (orders, claims, online, change of address): Elsevier Periodicals **Customer Service, 11830 Westline Industrial Drive, St. Louis, MO 63146. Tel: 1-800-654-2452 (U.S. and Canada); 314-453-7041 (outside U.S. and Canada). Fax: 314-453-5170. E-mail: journalscustomerservice-usa@elsevier.com (for print support); journalsonlinesupport-usa@elsevier.com (for online support).**

Reprints. For copies of 100 or more of articles in this publication, please contact the Commercial Reprints Department, Elsevier Inc., 360 Park Avenue South, New York, NY 10010-1710. Tel.: 212-633-3874; Fax: 212-633-3820; E-mail: reprints@elsevier.com.

Emergency Medicine Clinics of North America is covered in *MEDLINE/PubMed (Index Medicus), Current Contents/Clinical Medicine, EMBASE/Excerpta Medica, BIOSIS, SciSearch, CINAHL, ISI/BIOMED,* and *Research Alert.*

Contributors

CONSULTING EDITOR

AMAL MATTU, MD
Professor and Vice Chair of Education, Department of Emergency Medicine, University of Maryland School of Medicine, Baltimore, Maryland

EDITORS

LAURA J. BONTEMPO, MD, MEd
Assistant Professor, Department of Emergency Medicine, University of Maryland School of Medicine, Baltimore, Maryland

JAN SHOENBERGER, MD
Associate Professor of Clinical Emergency Medicine, Residency Program Director, Emergency Medicine, Keck School of Medicine of USC, University of Southern California, Los Angeles, California

AUTHORS

LAURA J. BONTEMPO, MD, MEd
Assistant Professor, Department of Emergency Medicine, University of Maryland School of Medicine, Baltimore, Maryland

STEVE CHUKWULEBE, MD
Resident Physician, Department of Emergency Medicine, Northwestern Medicine, Northwestern University Feinberg School of Medicine, Chicago, Illinois

STEPHANIE DIEBOLD, MD
Department of Emergency Medicine, Denver Health Hospital, Denver, Colorado

JASON FISCHEL, MD, MPH
EMS Division Chief, Department of Emergency Medicine, Norwalk Hospital, Norwalk, Connecticut

MEGAN LEIGH FIX, MD
Associate Professor, Division of Emergency Medicine, University of Utah, Salt Lake City, Utah

JEAN M. HAMMEL, MD, FACEP
Vice Chairperson, Department of Emergency Medicine, Norwalk Hospital, Norwalk, Connecticut

MAC HENRY, MD
Resident Physician, Alameda Health System, Highland Hospital, Oakland, California

H. GENE HERN, MD
Vice Chair of Education, Emergency Medicine, Associate Clinical Professor, University of California, San Francisco, Alameda Health System, Highland Hospital, Oakland, California

CHRISTOPHER HOGREFE, MD, FACEP
Assistant Professor, Departments of Emergency Medicine, Medicine - Sports Medicine, and Orthopaedic Surgery, Northwestern Medicine, Northwestern University Feinberg School of Medicine, Chicago, Illinois

MICHAEL KIEMENEY, MD
Assistant Professor, Loma Linda University School of Medicine, Loma Linda, California

MATTHEW R. KLEIN, MD, MPH
Instructor, Emergency Physician, Department of Emergency Medicine, Northwestern University, Chicago, Illinois

NEIL ALEXANDER KRULEWITZ, DO
Resident, Division of Emergency Medicine, University of Utah, Salt Lake City, Utah

RENJIE MICHAEL LI, MD
Loma Linda University Medical Center, Loma Linda, California

WILLIAM K. MALLON, MD, DTMH
Professor of Clinical Emergency Medicine, Department of Emergency Medicine, Director, Division of International EM, Stony Brook University (SUNY), Stony Brook, New York

SARA L. MANNING, MD
Assistant Professor, Department of Emergency Medicine, University of Maryland School of Medicine, Baltimore, Maryland

RODNEY OMRON, MD, MPH
Assistant Professor, Department of Emergency Medicine, Johns Hopkins School of Medicine, Baltimore, Maryland

MICHAEL OVERBECK, MD
Assistant Professor, Department of Emergency Medicine, University of Colorado School of Medicine, Denver, Colorado

LESLIE C. OYAMA, MD
Department of Emergency Medicine, University of California, San Diego, San Diego, California

JACOB SZMUILOWICZ, MD
Resident Physician, Department of Emergency Medicine, Kaiser Permanente, San Diego, California

BENJAMIN WYLER, MD, MPH, DTMH
Clinical Instructor, Department of Emergency Medicine, Stony Brook University (SUNY), Stony Brook, New York

RANDALL YOUNG, MD, MMM, FACEP
Clinical Faculty, Department of Emergency Medicine, Kaiser Permanente, San Diego, California

Contents

Infections of the ear are a common presentation to an acute care environment. In this article, the authors aim to summarize the most common presentations, and diagnostic and treatment options for typical infections of the ear. This article is geared toward the emergency physician, urgent care provider, and primary care provider who will likely be the initial evaluating and treating provider to assist them in determining what treatment modalities can be managed in a clinic and what needs to be referred for admission or specialty consultation.

This article summarizes the systematic assessment of the dizzy patient who presents with peripheral vertigo. It demonstrates the steps and tests necessary using the *Triage-Timing-Trigger– Test* (*Triage* + *TiTraTe*) method to accurately diagnose the underlying most probable cause while ruling out life-threatening causes. Using video support and just-in-time infographics, it demonstrates the Dix-Hallpike, Semont, Epley, and HINTS maneuvers.

Most anterior epistaxis originates primarily from the Kiesselbach plexus, whereas posterior epistaxis is less common and originates from branches of the sphenopalatine artery. Risk factors include local trauma, foreign body insertion, substance abuse, neoplasms, inherited bleeding diatheses, or acquired coagulopathies. Assessment of airway, breathing, and circulation precedes identification of bleeding source, pain control, and achieving hemostasis. Management options include topical vasoconstrictors, direct pressure, cautery, tranexamic acid, nasal tampons, Foley catheters, or surgical intervention. Specialty consultation may be pursued if interventions fail. Disposition is typically to home unless posterior epistaxis or significant comorbidities exist that warrant admission.

Rhinosinusitis affects many pediatric patients as well as 1 in 6 adults in any given year, resulting in ambulatory care, pediatric, and emergency department visits. Uncomplicated rhinosinusitis requires no imaging or testing and does not require antibiotic treatment. Using strict clinical diagnostic criteria may minimize unnecessary antibiotics. When indicated, amoxicillin with or without clavulanate for 5 to 10 days remains the first-line antibiotic, despite increasing incidence of staphylococcal sinusitis in the post-pneumococcal conjugate vaccine era. Emergency providers also need to recognize atypical cases in which uncommon but serious complications of sinusitis cause both morbidity and mortality.

of serious complications is low. These serious complications can, however, lead to significant morbidity and mortality and it is incumbent on the emergency provider to be prepared to deal with such tracheostomy-related emergencies. The greatest life threats to the tracheostomy patient are decannulation, obstruction, and hemorrhage. Other important but lower-acuity complications include tracheoesophageal fistula formation, tracheal stenosis, infection, and tracheocutaneous fistula formation.

EMERGENCY MEDICINE
CLINICS OF NORTH AMERICA

SERIES OF RELATED INTEREST

Critical Care Clinics
https://www.criticalcare.theclinics.com/
Otolaryngology Clinics
https://www.oto.theclinics.com/

THE CLINICS ARE NOW AVAILABLE ONLINE!
Access your subscription at:
www.theclinics.com

PROGRAM OBJECTIVE

The goal of *Emergency Medicine Clinics of North America* is to keep practicing emergency medicine physicians and emergency medicine residents up to date with current clinical practice in emergency medicine by providing timely articles reviewing the state of the art in patient care.

LEARNING OBJECTIVES

Upon completion of this activity, participants will be able to:

1. Review emergent infections of the ear, oropharynx and neck: presentation, diagnosis, and treatment options for emergency providers.
2. Recognize a systematic approach to the diagnosis and management of vertigo.
3. Discuss identification, etiology, and management of commonly observed conditions affecting the soft tissues of the mouth.

ACCREDITATION

The Elsevier Office of Continuing Medical Education (EOCME) is accredited by the Accreditation Council for Continuing Medical Education (ACCME) to provide continuing medical education for physicians.

The EOCME designates this enduring material for a maximum of 15 *AMA PRA Category 1 Credit*(s)™. Physicians should claim only the credit commensurate with the extent of their participation in the activity.

All other healthcare professionals requesting continuing education credit for this enduring material will be issued a certificate of participation.

DISCLOSURE OF CONFLICTS OF INTEREST

The EOCME assesses conflict of interest with its instructors, faculty, planners, and other individuals who are in a position to control the content of CME activities. All relevant conflicts of interest that are identified are thoroughly vetted by EOCME for fair balance, scientific objectivity, and patient care recommendations. EOCME is committed to providing its learners with CME activities that promote improvements or quality in healthcare and not a specific proprietary business or a commercial interest.

The planning committee, staff, authors and editors listed below have identified no financial relationships or relationships to products or devices they or their spouse/life partner have with commercial interest related to the content of this CME activity:

Laura J. Bontempo, MD, MEd; Steve Chukwulebe, MD; Stephanie Diebold, MD; Colleen Dietzler; Jason Fischel, MD, MPH; Megan Leigh Fix, MD; Jean M. Hammel, MD, FACEP; Mac Henry, MD; H. Gene Hern, MD; Christopher Hogrefe, MD, FACEP; Alison Kemp; Michael Kiemeney, MD; Matthew R. Klein, MD, MPH; Neil Alexander Krulewitz, DO; Renjie Michael Li, MD; William K. Mallon, MD, DTMH; Sara L. Manning, MD; Amal Mattu, MD; Rodney Omron, MD, MPH; Michael Overbeck, MD; Leslie C. Oyama, MD; Jan Shoenberger, MD; Jacob Szmuilowicz, MD; Vignesh Viswanathan; Benjamin Wyler, MD, MPH, DTMH; Randall Young, MD, MMM, FACEP.

UNAPPROVED/OFF-LABEL USE DISCLOSURE

The EOCME requires CME faculty to disclose to the participants:

1. When products or procedures being discussed are off-label, unlabelled, experimental, and/or investigational (not US Food and Drug Administration [FDA] approved); and
2. Any limitations on the information presented, such as data that are preliminary or that represent ongoing research, interim analyses, and/or unsupported opinions. Faculty may discuss information about pharmaceutical agents that is outside of FDA-approved labelling. This information is intended solely for CME and is not intended to promote off-label use of these medications. If you have any questions, contact the medical affairs department of the manufacturer for the most recent prescribing information.

TO ENROLL

To enroll in the *Emergency Medicine Clinics* Continuing Medical Education program, call customer service at 1-800-654-2452 or sign up online at http://www.theclinics.com/home/cme. The CME program is available to subscribers for an additional annual fee of $244 USD.

METHOD OF PARTICIPATION

In order to claim credit, participants must complete the following:

1. Complete enrolment as indicated above.
2. Read the activity.

3. Complete the CME Test and Evaluation. Participants must achieve a score of 70% on the test. All CME Tests and Evaluations must be completed online.

CME INQUIRIES/SPECIAL NEEDS

For all CME inquiries or special needs, please contact elsevierCME@elsevier.com.

Foreword

Ears, Nose, and Throat Emergencies

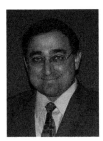

Amal Mattu, MD
Consulting Editor

I just recently completed the painful process of taking my second recertification examination in emergency medicine. The process of reviewing the entire core curriculum of our specialty every 10 years is always an eye-opening process, as I have a chance to review so many aspects of the specialty that have fallen from my "regularly used memory." In the process of this review, I became keenly aware once again of just how much of our specialty resides above the shoulders, yet outside the brain. Unbelievably, the ears, nose, mouth, and throat (the "head holes") account for the fourth most important organ system in terms of numbers of questions on the board exam, following cardiovascular, abdominal/gastrointestinal, and thoracic/respiratory. Then when I considered patients I see during a routine shift, it certainly corroborated the frequency of test questions related to the ears, nose, and throat (ENT). During my last shift, for example, I saw two patients with facial trauma from falls, a patient with epistaxis, a patient with a tracheostomy who was having dyspnea due to secretions, two patients with dizziness/vertigo, and a patient with a dental abscess. It was a good reminder of just how frequently patients present with ENT complaints, even if those presentations don't elicit the notoriety that strokes, heart attacks, and gunshot wounds do.

Two physicians who clearly know and understand the importance of ENT complaints are Drs Laura Bontempo and Jan Shoenberger. These emergency physicians, from opposite coasts, have taught extensively on these topics at continuing medical education courses, at board review courses, and in their own residency programs. They are well-recognized outstanding educators. They have teamed up to bring us a fantastic set of articles to teach us about the core curriculum and about cutting-edge care of patients with ENT emergencies. In order to do so, they have invited accomplished authors from both coasts in which they practice contribute. Significant, though appropriate, focus is placed in this issue on infections of the head, including the ear, sinuses, oropharynx, and neck. Soft tissue disorders are addressed as well as bony

Emerg Med Clin N Am 37 (2019) xi–xii
https://doi.org/10.1016/j.emc.2018.10.003
0733-8627/19/© 2018 Published by Elsevier Inc.

emed.theclinics.com

conditions such as fractures. Disorders of the mouth and teeth are discussed. Finally, two of the most challenging conditions in all of emergency medicine, vertigo and tracheostomy emergencies, are addressed in expert detail.

Drs Bontempo and Shoenberger and their authors are to be commended for their valuable contribution to the *Emergency Medicine Clinics of North America* series. This is must-reading for students and residents training in emergency medicine, and for any clinician working in either urgent or acute care settings. I anticipate referring to this issue many times between now and my next recertification exam in 10 years.

Amal Mattu, MD
Department of Emergency Medicine
University of Maryland School of Medicine
110 South Paca Street
6th Floor, Suite 200
Baltimore, MD 21201, USA

E-mail address:
amalmattu@comcast.net

Preface

Ear, Nose, and Throat Emergencies

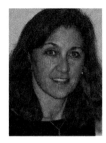 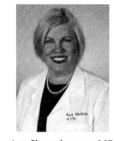

Laura J. Bontempo, MD, MEd   Jan Shoenberger, MD
Editors

The American Board of Emergency Medicine lists 30 specific Ear, Nose, and Throat disorders as well as five Otolaryngology-specific procedures in its 2016 Model of the Clinical Practice of Emergency Medicine. These disorders and their associated procedural skills range from critical in nature to lower acuity. As such, it is incumbent upon emergency providers to be prepared when these patients present for care. While specialty consultation with an otolaryngologist may be available at some centers, often timely access to such consultation is not possible.

Our goal in presenting this issue of *Emergency Medicine Clinics of North America* is to educate the emergency provider on the diagnosis and management of common and emergent ear, nose, and throat–related complaints. To the best of our knowledge, this is the first such publication to provide a focused review of these topics that is centered on evaluation, diagnosis, and treatment from the emergency medicine perspective.

The reader will notice that airway management and the creation of a surgical airway are not covered in this issue. We feel that there is adequate literature discussing these topics, and emergency physicians have many training opportunities in this aspect of our specialty. Instead, we opted to educate our readers on topics in which they may have less experience and fewer educational resources.

Of course, no such project can be completed without the effort of many individuals. We are reliant upon the work and dedication to detail of all our authors as well as the editorial staff of *Emergency Medicine Clinics of North America*. We also wish to offer our humble gratitude to Dr Amal Mattu for providing us this editorial opportunity.

Emerg Med Clin N Am 37 (2019) xiii–xiv
https://doi.org/10.1016/j.emc.2018.10.002
0733-8627/19/© 2018 Published by Elsevier Inc.

emed.theclinics.com

We hope that you find this information useful and that it increases your comfort and skills when caring for your patients. Thank you for reading our work.

Laura J. Bontempo, MD, MEd
Department of Emergency Medicine
University of Maryland School of Medicine
110 South Paca Street
6th Floor, Suite 200
Baltimore, MD 21201, USA

Jan Shoenberger, MD
Clinical Emergency Medicine
Keck School of Medicine
University of Southern California
1975 Zonal Avenue
Los Angeles, CA 90033, USA

E-mail addresses:
Lbontempo@som.umaryland.edu (L.J. Bontempo)
janshoenberger@me.com (J. Shoenberger)

Erratum

The following errors were found in the article, "Pediatric Sepsis" by Melanie K. Prusa-kowski and Audrey P. Chen in the *Severe Sepsis Care in the Emergency Department* issue of *Emergency Medicine Clinics of North America* (February 2017, Volume 35, Issue 1, p1-240):

On Page 133, in the section on Catecholamine-resistant shock, Waterhouse-Frider-ichen should be Waterhouse-Friderichsen.

On page 134, in Table 4, in the row for Burn victims, under typical pathogens, the second line should be Staphylococcus aureus instead of Streptococcus aureus.

https://doi.org/10.1016/j.emc.2018.10.001
0733-8627/19/© 2016 Elsevier Inc. All rights reserved.
emed.theclinics.com

Infections of the Ear

Jacob Szmuilowicz, MD, Randall Young, MD, MMM*

KEYWORDS

• Ear infections • Summary • Review

KEY POINTS

- This article is a concise review of common infections of the ear and recommended diagnostic and treatment options for emergency providers.
- Infections of the ear are summarized by their different anatomic compartments (outer, middle, and inner).
- Common treatments and potential pitfalls for the treating emergency provider are discussed.

INTRODUCTION

Infections of the ear can be broken down into 3 distinct areas, the outer, the middle, and the inner ear. Because affected patients present with different complaints, a careful history and physical examination are very important. Outer ear infections are referred to as otitis externa; middle ear infections are referred to as otitis media, and inner ear infections are referred to as otitis interna, but are most generally thought of as labyrinthitis or neuronitis.

OUTER EAR INFECTIONS

Outer ear infections are described as infections ranging from the outside surface of the head to the eardrum or tympanic membrane (TM). The authors cover 3 basic types of outer ear infections, otitis externa (swimmer's ear), perichondritis, and malignant otitis externa.

Otitis Externa

Commonly referred to as swimmer's ear, the term can be a bit misleading because the patient does not need to swim in order to be afflicted by this infection. Most often otitis externa is caused by a bacterial infection, but in some cases, fungi can also cause this infection. Risk factors for otitis externa include the following: swimmers with risk

Disclosure Statement: Nothing to disclose, no conflicts to report.
Department of Emergency Medicine, Kaiser Permanente, 4647 Zion Avenue, San Diego, CA 92120, USA
* Corresponding author.
E-mail address: rjyoungmd@kaiser-ed.com

amplified by the use of earplugs, chronic dermatitis conditions (eczema, psoriasis, and so forth), use of cotton swabs to clean their ears or those who use earplugs, and use of potentially caustic irritants near their ears (hair dyes, hair sprays, and so forth).

The diagnosis of otitis externa is made by a careful history and physical examination. Patients will complain of pain with movement or palpation of the outer ear or itching of the ear canal. A clinician performing an examination should pay attention to pain with manipulation of the pinna or auricle. Examination of the auditory canal via an otoscope will demonstrate an edematous and erythematous auditory canal sometimes lined with pus or debris. The examination should ensure that the TM is intact because this would alter the treatment regimen. When the findings occur in an elderly diabetic or other immunocompromised patient, malignant otitis externa must be considered.

The most common causative organisms of otitis externa are *Pseudomonas aeruginosa* and *Staphylococcus aureus*. Other organisms, however, can be involved, such as other bacteria, viruses, and fungi. Obtaining a culture may be considered and would be helpful if the initial treatment results in failure. In patients with a history of repeated otitis externa treated with antibiotic drops, fungal infections should strongly be considered. The most common fungal infections include Aspergillus and Candida. In these cases, diagnosis can be made by careful examination of the ear to look for black fungal colonies (aspergillus) or white fungal colonies (candida).

With an intact TM, the recommended treatment of otitis externa involves the use of topical drops, usually a topical antibiotic that may be combined with a steroid or a 2% acetic acid otic solution. The typical antibiotic component of drops is most commonly a quinolone or aminoglycoside, although some formularies may prefer a neomycin or Polymyxin-B formulation. With a ruptured TM, ofloxacin otic drops[1] or oral antibiotics are the recommended treatment. By slightly lowering the pH of the external ear canal with a 2% acetic acid solution, the environment is altered, making it inhospitable to typical bacterial growth. The possible risk, however, is that by lowering the pH, the slightly caustic nature of the solution can lead to trauma in the ear canal, thereby increasing risk of an infection by the decreased barrier of the epithelium. Patients rarely require systemic treatment with oral or intravenous (IV) antibiotics; however, consideration should be given to patients with a toxic appearance or those with a known immunodeficiency or who are immunosuppressed.

Key points

- Diagnosis of acute otitis externa is made by careful history and physical examination. Emergency providers should have a high level of suspicion in those who are at risk, such as swimmers, those with chronic dermatitis, or those with recent trauma.
- Treatment depends on whether the TM is intact.
- Antibiotic drops with or without a corticosteroid are the mainstay of treatment, but other treatments may involve a 2% acetic acid solution.
- Systemic antibiotic therapy is rarely required.

Perichondritis

Perichondritis is an infection of the cartilage of the outer aspect (auricle) of the ear. Perichondritis is often caused by piercings, surgery, burns, or ear trauma or overlying skin infections. This can be complicated by patients with immunodeficiencies or diabetes. Patients will present with complaints of redness, pain, and swelling around the auricle. In early stages, simple induration may be found, whereas in later stages, fluctuance may be palpated. In these later stages, there is often an accumulation of pus under the surface that must be drained for infection control. If there is a foreign body such as a piercing that could be seeding the infection, it must also be removed. Appropriate treatment involves both incision and drainage and antibiotic therapy. As with other types of abscesses, antibiotic therapy alone is not sufficient once this infection has organized. The most common microbial species isolated from a perichondrial infection is *P aeruginosa*.[2] Antibiotic treatment choice has centered on the use of fluoroquinolones with ciprofloxacin oral treatment as the mainstay. Unfortunately, because *P aeruginosa* is one of the notorious SPACE organisms (*Serratia*, *P aeruginosa*, *Acinetobacter*, *Citrobacter*, *Enterobacter cloacea*), it is known to rapidly develop antibiotic resistance, even against fluoroquinolones.[3] Frequent follow-up is imperative, and parenteral antibiotic therapy may be required. Treatment of perichondritis can be very challenging and should not be considered complete in a single emergency department (ED) visit. The patient should be referred to an otolaryngologist because the potential complication of unsuccessful treatment can lead to lifelong disfigurement.

Potential complications of perichondritis include reaccumulation of the abscess or formation of a seroma in the potential space caused by the previous abscess and/or cartilaginous destruction of the auricle caused by pressure against the cartilage resulting in permanent deformity of the ear (cauliflower ear).

Key points

- Diagnosis of perichondritis is made by history and physical examination. Emergency providers should have a high level of suspicion in patients who have had recent ear trauma.
- Abscess formation is a common complication and can lead to lifelong disfigurement if not appropriately drained.
- Oral, or in some cases, IV antibiotics, are the mainstay of therapy. The most common causative organism is *P aeruginosa*.
- Referral to an otolaryngologist should always be considered because management of a cartilaginous infection is challenging.

Malignant Otitis Externa

Malignant otitis externa is a very rare complication of the spread of otitis externa into the mastoid and/or temporal bone causing osteomyelitis. The most common organism that causes malignant otitis externa is *P aeruginosa*.[4] This complication does not usually occur in those who are otherwise young and immunocompetent. It should be suspected in those who are elderly or immunocompromised, such as patients with AIDS or a relative immunocompromised state, such as diabetes or patients on chronic steroids or immunosuppressive medications.

Presenting symptoms of malignant otitis externa are headache with otalgia, sometimes with vertigo and decreased hearing. Physical examination reveals an examination that is similar to what would be expected for a severe case of otitis externa, often with purulent or foul-smelling drainage. In addition, there will likely be pain on bony palpation of the mastoid or adjacent areas of the skull.

Confirmation of the diagnosis of malignant otitis externa is made by MRI or computed tomographic (CT) scanning. Additional laboratory tests that can be useful not only in diagnosis but also in monitoring of treatment include a complete blood count and inflammatory markers, erythrocyte sedimentation rate, and C-reactive protein. Upon confirmation of the diagnosis of malignant otitis externa, immediate consultation with otolaryngology should be obtained.

Treatment of malignant otitis externa typically requires prolonged IV antibiotic therapy, often extending for at least 6 weeks, strict glucose control, if applicable, and hyperbaric oxygen treatment may be considered. Necrotic tissue within the external auditory canal will likely require frequent debridement; however, bony resection is rarely indicated. Despite aggressive treatment, mortality in malignant otitis externa is still 10% to 20%.[4]

Key points

- Malignant otitis externa is a rare complication of otitis externa with a very high mortality. It should be considered in elderly diabetic and immunocompromised patients.
- Accurate diagnosis requires advanced imaging with either MRI or CT scan.
- The most common causative organism is typically *P aeruginosa*, and initial treatment is with IV fluoroquinolones.
- With a confirmed diagnosis or a high level of suspicion, otolaryngology should be immediately consulted and the patient should be hospitalized.

MIDDLE EAR INFECTIONS

The middle ear is defined by the TM and the adjacent air-containing chamber that houses the 3 auditory ossicles. Sound waves enter the external ear and are funneled to the middle ear, where the vibrations are then transmitted and amplified via the TM and auditory ossicle to the inner ear. The middle ear chamber additionally communicates with the eustachian tube and the mastoid air spaces. This section discusses infections of the middle ear, primarily otitis media, and its associated infectious complications, including mastoiditis and myringitis.

Otitis Media

Infection or inflammation of the middle ear is broadly known as otitis media. When symptom onset occurs rapidly, it is called acute otitis media (AOM). Although AOM is seen in both adults and children, it primarily seen in the pediatrics population. Children are thought to be more susceptible to AOM because of their unique anatomy. Shorter, immature, and more horizontally oriented eustachian tubes produce a more favorable environment for infections.

AOM most commonly occurs in association with, or soon after, a viral upper respiratory infection (URI). Inflammation obstructs flow through the eustachian tube and creates conditions favorable for middle ear infections. *Streptococcus pneumoniae*, nontypeable *Haemophilus influenzae*, and *Moraxella catarrhalis* are the most commonly identified bacterial organisms.[5,6] *S aureus* and *P aeruginosa* have also been known to cause AOM, but are generally more often associated with chronic otitis media.[5,7]

The diagnosis of AOM is largely based on the obtained history and physical examination. Patients presenting to the ED frequently describe a few days of URI symptoms or a recently resolved URI, followed by sudden onset, worsening otalgia. Fever, conductive hearing loss, and otorrhea may also be reported. Otorrhea should alert the clinician to inspect for perforation of the TM. Regarding the pediatric population, patients may be more irritable and fussy than usual. Holding, tugging, or rubbing the affected ear is also commonly reported. On examination, otoscopic visualization shows a retracted or bulging TM, and there is impaired TM mobility on pneumatic otoscopy. In addition, the TM may be erythematous from inflammation or yellow or white secondary to a middle ear effusion. A complete examination of the cranial nerves should also be performed because of their proximity to the middle ear, because many severe complications of AOM extend beyond the confines of the middle ear chamber.

Of note, otitis media with effusion (OME) is a common sequela of AOM, but it is not considered an infection. OME presents with ear discomfort, sensation of ear fullness, or decreased hearing without pain. Symptoms may persist for weeks to months. On examination, patients may have a middle ear effusion with little inflammatory changes and an immobile TM on pneumatic otoscopy. As OME is not an infection, antibiotics are not helpful, and most cases resolve spontaneously, generally without requiring treatment, and without complications. Watchful waiting is the most common approach to managing this condition.

Complications from AOM are relatively infrequent, but should be considered when managing any patient with a presentation suggestive of otitis media. The most common complication is perforation of the TM. This is caused by increased pressure produced by fluid accumulation in the middle ear. Patients may describe ear pain, hearing loss, otorrhea, tinnitus, or vertigo. Management consists of oral and topical antibiotics. The same oral antibiotics used to cover the initial AOM infection, as discussed later in this section, are appropriate, and topical antibiotics, such as ofloxacin, may also be included. In most cases, TM perforation heals within a few weeks without needing additional intervention; however, chronic perforation may require otolaryngology evaluation. Bacterial translocation to adjacent structures may cause subsequent infection of the labyrinth or mastoid air cells, resulting in acute labyrinthitis or acute mastoiditis, respectively. The most severe complications are seen when there is intracranial extension of the infection. Although extremely rare, meningitis, brain abscess, and lateral sinus thrombosis are known intracranial complications of otitis media. Any signs of facial nerve paralysis or other focal neurologic findings in the setting of an ear infection should be evaluated with advanced imaging, such as CT or MRI, and emergent otolaryngology or neurosurgery consultation.

Regarding treatment options, management of the symptoms associated with AOM often provides patients with satisfactory relief. AOM is often painful, and otalgia should always be treated adequately. Oral analgesics, including acetaminophen and/or ibuprofen, are frequently recommended. Acetaminophen is additionally encouraged for the febrile patient. Remember to use weight-based dosing for pediatric patients. Topical intranasal vasoconstrictors, such as phenylephrine drops, may improve eustachian tube function, and systemic decongestants, such as pseudoephedrine, may also provide benefit. Narcotic pain medications are rarely needed and should be used judiciously and only in severe cases. Topical analgesics, including antipyrine and benzocaine otic drops, have also been suggested, but in 2015, the Food and Drug Administration stopped the sales of ear-drop medications containing benzocaine and antipyrine, claiming that these medications have not been evaluated for safety, effectiveness, and quality.[8]

Although the symptomatic management of AOM is largely the same for most patients, the approach to antibiotic treatments differs depending on the patient's age. Treatment guidelines for pediatric patients recommend a "wait-and-see" approach in select children with nonsevere symptoms. This includes children ages 6 to 23 months with unilateral AOM, or patients 24 months and older with either unilateral or bilateral AOM.[9,10] In this population, AOM often resolves spontaneously and without complication,[11] thus avoiding the potential side effects associated with antibiotics and the possible proliferation of drug-resistant organisms. The "wait-and-see" treatment option includes appropriate analgesics, joint decision making, and education with the patient's parents, close physician follow-up, and a plan to start antibiotics in 48 to 72 hours if symptoms worsen or fail to improve (delayed prescription).[9,10] In children who do not qualify for the "wait-and-see" approach, the recommended first-line treatment is amoxicillin 40 to 45 mg/kg twice a day. Treatment for 5 to

7 days is suggested for children 2 years or older with nonsevere symptoms or those who fail the "wait-and-see" period, whereas 10 days of therapy is advised for younger patients or any patient with evidence of more severe signs or symptoms.[9,10] In adult patients, the "wait-and-see" approach to treatment has not been evaluated, and initial treatment with antibiotics is considered the standard of practice. Similarly, amoxicillin is also considered first-line therapy, with dosing of 500 mg every 12 hours for mild or moderate symptoms, and 875 mg every 12 hours or 500 mg every 8 hours for more severe cases.[12] For penicillin-allergic patients, alternatives include cefdinir, cefuroxime, cefpodoxime, or ceftriaxone. In addition, if the patient does not seem to be improving after 48 to 72 hours of initial therapy, alternatives include amoxicillin-clavulanate, levofloxacin, or moxifloxacin.

Most patients will see improvement within 24 to 48 hours of starting appropriate treatment. As long as there is consistent symptomatic improvement, patients may be managed in the outpatient setting with close follow-up to assess for improvement and treatment efficacy. If the patient is not improving, it may be appropriate to adjust the antibiotic regimen. Any patient that appears septic or develops complications may benefit from inpatient admission for IV antibiotics or specialist consultation with otolaryngology.

Key points

- AOM is typically a pediatric diagnosis, but can also be seen in adults.
- AOM is diagnosed based on careful history and physical examination, including otoscopic evaluation.
- Complications of AOM are infrequent, but should always be considered. Evidence of persistent symptoms, severe infection, or abnormal focal neurologic findings should be further evaluated with specialist consultation.
- Uncomplicated AOM in children may be treated with analgesics and the "wait-and-see" approach to antibiotics; however, close outpatient physician follow-up should be ensured.
- The "wait-and-see" approach has not been adequately studied in adults, and AOM should be treated with appropriate antibiotics.

Mastoiditis

Mastoiditis generally develops as a complication of AOM when infection and inflammation of the inner ear spread to the adjacent mastoid air cells. The diagnosis is frequently made clinically, based on the history and physical examination. Patients present with a similar constellation of symptoms than with AOM, including otalgia, fever, otorrhea, but mastoiditis is additionally classically characterized by postauricular erythema, edema, and tenderness, with protrusion of the auricle.[13] If there is any doubt of the diagnosis, or concern for additional adjacent soft tissue involvement, contrast CT or MRI imaging of the mastoid may be obtained. As mastoiditis is considered an invasive infection, IV antibiotics and inpatient hospital admission are generally recommended. Early specialist consultation should also be obtained as myringotomy, tympanostomy tube placement, and in severe cases, mastoidectomy may be required. Antibiotic regimens should be appropriately selected to cover for the most typically responsible pathogens, including S pneumoniae, Streptococcus pyogenes, S aureus, and P aeruginosa.[14]

Key points

- Mastoiditis is a known complication of AOM due to bacterial translocation to the mastoid air cells.

- Patients classically present with postauricular erythema, edema, and auricular protrusion in the setting of an AOM infection.
- CT or MRI imaging may be helpful in confirming the diagnosis or evaluating for other possible complications.
- Management consists of IV antibiotics and otolaryngology consultation.

Myringitis

Another condition associated with otitis media is bullous myringitis. Inflammation causes blistering and formation of bullae on the TM and the inner auditory canal. Patients typically present with severe otalgia, but can develop hearing loss or fever. As the bullae rupture, patients can also experience otorrhea. Diagnosis is made on physical examination of the TM and ear canal with direct otoscopic visualization of the lesions. Bullous myringitis is caused by the typical AOM organisms; thus, management is the same. Treatment includes oral and possibly topical analgesics and antibiotics. Severe cases may require otolaryngology consultation for procedural rupturing of the lesions.

Key points

- Bullous myringitis is associated with AOM and leads to blisters or bullae forming on the TM or auditory canal secondary to inflammation.
- Bullous myringitis is associated with otorrhea, which occurs when the lesions rupture.
- Diagnosis is made on physical examination with direct otoscopic visualization of the lesions.
- Treatment is identical to that of the underlying AOM infection.

INNER EAR INFECTIONS

The inner ear is largely made up of 2 structures, the vestibular system and the cochlea. The vestibular system, comprising the semicircular canals and the vestibule, is responsible for balance, while the cochlea converts mechanical vibrations into electrical signals to the brain, which makes it possible to perceive and hear sound. Although frequently thought of as similar diseases, labyrinthitis and vestibular neuronitis are the most common infections of the inner ear.

Labyrinthitis

As its name suggests, labyrinthitis is an infection of the labyrinth. This structure becomes infected by bacterial translocation into the inner ear. Most commonly, this occurs secondary to AOM but has also been associated with meningitis, mastoiditis, cholesteatoma, or after traumatic fracture of the labyrinth, which allows seeding of infectious organisms. Patients typically present with some combination of vertigo, nystagmus, or hearing loss together with evidence of an AOM infection. Patients may also experience fever, otalgia, nausea, vomiting, or tinnitus. Although the diagnosis is often clinical, based on history, symptoms, and physical examination findings, CT or MRI imaging may be useful to confirm the diagnosis or evaluate for complications. Because of the inner ear's proximity to the central nervous system, treatment often consists of inpatient hospital admission and IV antibiotics that provide adequate coverage for meningitis, commonly ceftriaxone 50 to 100 mg/kg IV daily up to a maximum of 2 g. If this diagnosis is suspected, early otolaryngologist consultation is recommended because the patient may benefit from myringotomy or mastoidectomy in more severe cases.

Key points

- Labyrinthitis generally presents with vertigo and hearing loss in the setting of concurrent or recent AOM; however, it can also be associated with other infectious or traumatic causes.
- Labyrinthitis can have severe complications due to its relative proximity to the central nervous system.
- CT or MRI may be useful for ruling out other causes of vertigo.
- Management consists of IV antibiotics and otolaryngologist consultation.

Vestibular Neuronitis

Although often considered synonymous with labyrinthitis, vestibular neuronitis has a few important distinctions. Patients with vestibular neuronitis present with sudden, severe vertigo in the setting of an ongoing or recent upper respiratory viral infection, and symptoms may persist for several days to a few weeks. They may additionally have associated nausea, vomiting, and horizontal nystagmus. The diagnosis is made clinically, based on history and physical examination; however, additional testing may be needed to exclude other causes of vertigo. In contrast to labyrinthitis, these patients do not experience tinnitus or hearing loss. As it is primarily considered to be due to a viral cause, the infection is self-limiting, and treatment consists of symptomatic management. In addition to traditional antiemetics, options for treatment include medications with antiemetic properties, including anticholinergics, antihistamines, or benzodiazepines. There is insufficient evidence to suggest improvement with corticosteroid medications.[15]

Key points

- Vestibular neuronitis is often synonymous with labyrinthitis, but is generally thought to be associated with a viral, rather than bacterial, cause.
- Patients also present with sudden, severe vertigo, but as opposed to labyrinthitis, do not experience tinnitus or hearing loss.
- Because the cause is ultimately due to a viral infection, management is symptomatic.

REFERENCES

1. Simpson KL, Markman A. Ofloxacin otic solution: a review of its use in the management of ear infections. Drugs 1999;58(3):509–31.
2. Prasad HK, Sreedharan S, Prasad HS, et al. Perichondritis of the auricle and its management. J Laryngol Otol 2007;121(6):530–4.
3. Wu DC, Chan WW, Metelitsa AI, et al. Pseudomonas skin infection: clinical features, epidemiology, and management. Am J Clin Dermatol 2011;12(3):157–69.
4. Bhandary S, Karki P, Sinha BK. Malignant otitis externa: a review. Pac Health Dialog 2002;9(1):64–7.
5. Ruohola A, Meurman O, Nikkari S, et al. Microbiology of acute otitis media in children with tympanostomy tubes: prevalences of bacteria and viruses. Clin Infect Dis 2006;43(11):1417–22.
6. Pumarola F, Marès J, Losada I, et al. Microbiology of bacteria causing recurrent acute otitis media (AOM) and AOM treatment failure in young children in Spain: shifting pathogens in the post-pneumococcal conjugate vaccination era. Int J Pediatr Otorhinolaryngol 2013;77(8):1231–6.

7. Lin YS, Lin LC, Lee FP, et al. The prevalence of chronic otitis media and its complication rates in teenagers and adult patients. Otolaryngol Head Neck Surg 2009;140(2):165–70.
8. US Food and Drug Administration. FDA: use only approved prescription ear drops. Available at: https://www.fda.gov/ForConsumers/ConsumerUpdates/ucm453087. htm. Accessed June 8, 2018.
9. Lieberthal AS, Carroll AE, Chonmaitree T, et al. The diagnosis and management of acute otitis media. Pediatrics 2013;131(3):e964–99.
10. Harmes KM, Blackwood RA, Burrows HL, et al. Otitis media: diagnosis and treatment. Am Fam Physician 2013;88(7):435–40.
11. Marchetti F, Ronfani L, Nibali SC, et al. Delayed prescription may reduce the use of antibiotics for acute otitis media: a prospective observational study in primary care. Arch Pediatr Adolesc Med 2005;159(7):679–84.
12. Limb CJ, Lustig LR, Klein JO, et al. Acute otitis media in adults. Available at: https://www. uptodate.com/contents/acute-otitis-media-in- adults. Accessed May 25, 2018.
13. Hosmer K. Ear disorders. In: Tintinalli JE, Stapczynski JS, Ma OJ, et al, editors. Tintinalli's emergency medicine: a comprehensive study guide. 8th edition. New York: McGraw-Hill Education LLC; 2011. Available at: https://accessemergencymedicine. mhmedical.com/content.aspx?sectionid=109387021&bookid=1658&Resultclick=2. Accessed May 25, 2018.
14. Laulajainen-Hongisto A, Saat R, Lempinen L, et al. Bacteriology in relation to clinical findings and treatment of acute mastoiditis in children. Int J Pediatr Otorhinolaryngol 2014;78(12):2072–8.
15. Fishman JM, Burgess C, Waddell A. Corticosteroids for the treatment of idiopathic acute vestibular dysfunction (vestibular neuritis). Cochrane Database Syst Rev 2011;(11):CD008607.

Peripheral Vertigo

Rodney Omron, MD, MPH

KEYWORDS

- Peripheral vertigo • Hints • Head impulse test • Dix-hallpike • Epley • Nystagmus
- Test of skew

KEY POINTS

- A systematic approach to the management of vertigo is more accurate than subcategorizing patients based on the question, "What do you mean by dizzy?".
- Use the Dix-Hallpike to diagnose posterior canal–triggered episodic vertigo then treat with an Epley or Semont maneuver.
- Use HINTS + hearing loss to diagnose acute vestibular neuritis.
- Reserve MRI and central nervous system workup for groups that neither have benign paroxysmal positional vertigo nor acute vestibular neuritis based on *Tri*age, *Ti*ming, *Tr*iggers, and *Ta*rgeted *E*xam + *Tests* (*Triage + TiTraTe + Tests*).
- Never perform computed tomography for dizziness unless there is a possible risk of intracranial bleeding, such as patients on anticoagulation or trauma, although posterior fossa hemorrhages usually present with headache and changes in mental status.

INTRODUCTION

Dizziness is a common chief complaint resulting in about 4% of all emergency department (ED) visits.[1] Defining dizziness by the subcategories of vertigo and lightheadedness offers no benefit in diagnosing the underlying disease.[2,3] Instead asking questions about associated factors (triage), timing, and triggers and then completing focused physical examination tests based on the responses have been shown to be more accurate than performing advanced imaging such as computed tomography (CT) or MRI in making the correct diagnosis and ruling out life-threatening causes.[4]

Reliance on advanced imaging without a systematic problem-based history and physical in the evaluation of the dizzy patient has been shown to increase length of stay,[5] increase cost of care,[6] and has falsely reassured providers that a life-threatening cause has been ruled out when it has not.[6] Often times, a normal head CT scan is done to evaluate for intracranial hemorrhage, which has little diagnostic yield in an isolated dizzy patient.[6] Furthermore, causes such as benign paroxysmal

Disclosure Statement: The author has no financial interests to disclose.
Department of Emergency Medicine, Johns Hopkins Medical School, Johns Hopkins University School of Medicine, 733 North Broadway, Baltimore, MD 21205, USA
E-mail address: romron1@jhmi.edu

Emerg Med Clin N Am 37 (2019) 11–28
https://doi.org/10.1016/j.emc.2018.09.004
emed.theclinics.com

positional vertigo (BPPV) cannot be diagnosed with advanced imaging and is completely reliant on physical examination findings to accurately diagnose and treat. If left untreated, there is a considerable morbidity associated with peripheral vertigo in time missed from work,[7] with a 6.5-fold increase in risk of falls[6] and high risk of reoccurrence (46% vs 20%; $P = .002$).[6] This article discusses the evaluation and treatment of the most common causes of peripheral vertigo. For more information on the assessment and management of central vertigo please see Emergency Neurootology: Diagnosis and Management of Acute Dizziness and Vertigo, which is an emergency-focused clinics edition dedicated to the complete evaluation of the dizzy patient.[8] Most of this article is a summarized adaptation of that edition and most of the graphics are also from that edition.

NEW DIAGNOSTIC APPROACH

The differential diagnosis for dizziness is broad with no one cause accounting for more than 10% of ED presentations.[1] Because there is not one predominate diagnosis, an algorithmic approach seeking high-risk low-frequency causes such as stroke while ruling in likely causes such as BPPV is preferred to grouping cases based on the question "What do you mean by dizzy?".[2] Some rare diseases need to be considered in *every* dizzy patient even if a clinician will only personally see a few of these rare presentations in their career. Without a systematic approach or direct feedback about every dizzy patient that is seen, chances are that misdiagnosis will go undetected and the clinician will have little opportunity for recalibration. For example, posterior stroke is misdiagnosed 59% of the time in the ED,[9] leading to an absolute number of up to 75,000 patients harmed per year[9] despite the low individual number of cases

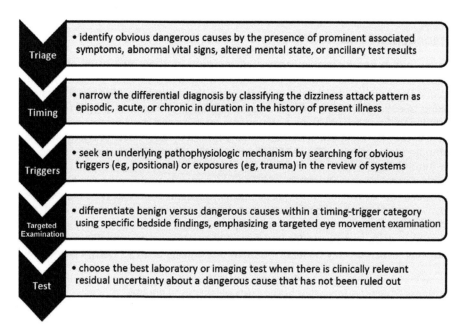

Fig. 1. The triage–TiTrATE–test approach to diagnosing dizziness and vertigo. The TiTrATE acronym stands for timing, triggers, and targeted examinations. (*Adapted from* Neuro-ophthalmology virtual education library. Available at: https://collections.lib.utah.edu/ark:/ 87278/s6tm7cr7. Accessed October 11, 2018; with permission.)[10]

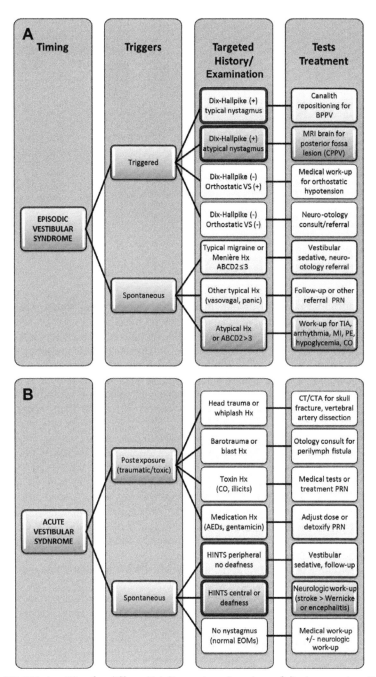

Fig. 2. TiTrATE algorithm for differential diagnosis and workup of dizziness and vertigo. The TiTrATE algorithm divides acute dizziness and vertigo into 4 key categories: (*A*) t-EVS and s-EVS forms of EVS and (*B*) t-AVS and s-AVS forms of AVS. Each syndrome determines a targeted bedside examination, differential diagnosis, and tests, regardless of symptom type (vertigo, presyncope, unsteadiness, or nonspecific dizziness). Some steps may occur after the ED visit, as part of follow-up or during inpatient hospital admission. Box color in the

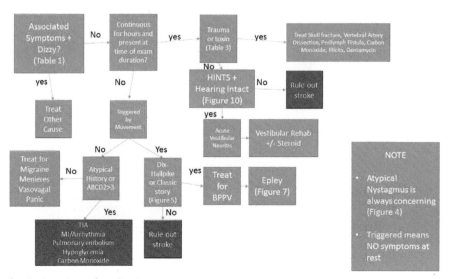

Fig. 3. Overview of evaluation.

seen per individual clinician career. If one does not consider these rare but life-threatening diagnoses or simply have feedback on mistakes, a clinician may be unknowingly discharging patients with life-threatening causes of dizziness despite years of clinical practice. The Triage– Titrate model of diagnosing the emergency dizzy patient is a systematic way to approach the dizzy patient with proven efficacy.[2] Instead of incorporating the review of systems at the end of the patient evaluation when it is an afterthought, this new approach starts with looking at associated symptoms that suggest neurologic conditions that should not be missed. This is the *Triage* component of the approach (**Fig. 1**).

After *Triage* is performed, then next step is *TiTrATE + Tests*: (*Ti*ming, *Tr*iggers *A*nd *T*argeted *E*xam + *Tests* [**Fig. 2**]). Timing classifies the disease processes into episodic versus continuous. Triggers further seek to find the underlying causes by looking for physical examination findings (eg, Dix-Hallpike) or review of symptoms questions (eg, history of trauma). One then performs a targeted examination based on these findings and ancillary tests are based on that examination. The combination of these information allows the clinician to base imaging, such as CT and MRI, on specific triage, timing, triggers, and examination to maximize the testing utility and minimize unnecessary tests (see **Fig. 2**).

For an interactive online infographic to evaluate the dizzy patient, see the following url: https://connect.johnshopkins.edu/dizzyinfo.

This infographic contains a guide map for just-in-time reminders with in-depth hyperlinks that refer you to teaching videos and diagrams (**Fig. 3**). Each box in the graph will represent a section below.

Targeted and Tests columns denotes risk of a dangerous disorder (*red*, high; *yellow*, intermediate; and *green*, low). Bold outlines denote evidence-based, targeted eye examinations that discriminate between benign and dangerous causes. AED, antiepileptic drug; CO, carbon monoxide; EOM, extraocular movement; Hx, history; MI, myocardial infarction; PE, pulmonary embolus; PRN, pro re nata (as needed); VS, vital signs. (*Adapted from* Neuro-ophthalmology virtual education library. Available at: https://collections.lib.utah.edu/ark:/87278/s6tm7cr7. Accessed October 11, 2018; with permission.)[10]

Associated
Symptoms +
Dizzy? (Click
to see)

TRIAGE (ASSOCIATED SYMPTOMS IN ADDITION TO CHIEF COMPLAINT OF DIZZINESS)

Seeking associated factors in addition to the chief complaint of "Dizzy" is known as the "*Triage*" step in determining the underlying cause. Diseases such as alcoholism, pulmonary embolism, myocardial infarction, carbon monoxide poisoning, hypertension, acute coronary syndrome, and toxic levels of medications can mimic a vestibular cause (**Box 1**). In the spirit of the flipped classroom please see the following cases that are presented as unknowns with associated symptoms in the dizzy patient: https://connect.johnshopkins.edu/vertigooverview.

Box 1
Dizzy + associated symptoms, signs, or laboratory results

Altered Mental Status—seizure, alcohol, carbon monoxide, Wernicke, stroke, hypertension, encephalitis

Loss of Consciousness—acute coronary syndrome, seizure, aortic dissection, pulmonary embolism, stroke, vasovagal, subarachnoid hemorrhage, hypovolemia, arrhythmias

Neck Pain—Craniocervical dissection

Chest/Back Pain—acute coronary syndrome, aortic dissection

Abdominal Pain—ruptured ectopic, aortic dissection

Dyspnea—pulmonary embolism, pneumonia, anemia

Palpitations—arrhythmia, vasovagal, panic attack, hyperthyroid bleeding/fluid loss

Meds

Fever—mastoiditis, meningitis, encephalitis, infection

Abnormal Glucose—hypoglycemia, diabetic ketoacidosis

Adapted from Newman-Toker DE, Edlow JA. TiTrATE: a novel, evidence-based approach to diagnosing acute dizziness and vertigo. Neurol Clin 2015;33(3):577–99.

Continuous
for hours and
present at
time of exam
duration?

Triggered
by
Movement

Trauma
or toxin
(Click to
see)

TIMING AND TRIGGERS

The clinician must identify the duration of the dizziness episodes, whether they are episodic or continuous and what (if anything) triggers the episodes. There are 6 vestibular syndromes based on timing and triggers (**Table 1**). It is important to understand that any type of dizziness gets worse with position change. There must be no symptoms present without the trigger to diagnose triggered episodic vestibular syndrome (t-EVS). In case of BPPV, there must be no vertigo present unless the head is moved, although they may still have residual nondizzy symptoms such as nausea. Acute vestibular syndrome (AVS) can be triggered by a toxin or trauma (triggered acute vestibular syndrome [t-AVS]) or spontaneously (spontaneous s-AVS). This article discusses causes that are only associated with peripheral vertigo (t-EVS vs s-EVS, t-AVS vs s-AVS). To learn more about the central and chronic causes (t-CVS and s-CVS) look toward the comprehensive review at the following reference.[8]

New-Onset Episodic Vestibular Syndrome

EVS is defined as seconds, minutes, or hours of vertigo. It usually has a very short duration of less than 30 seconds. Relapsing symptoms that last for weeks are not considered new onset and therefore fall in the chronic category.[2]

New-Onset Triggered Episodic Vestibular Syndrome

This is a vestibular syndrome that is triggered by something. It must not be present without the trigger and must be initiated with the trigger. The trigger is often change in head position but may be a loud sound or Valsalva.[2] The physical examination should be directed at demonstrating the underlying physical finding for different

Table 1
Timing and triggers of 6 vestibular syndromes

Name	Symptoms
Triggered episodic vestibular syndrome (t-EVS)	Brief, event triggered discrete episodes lasting <24 h then resolving before the next episode
Spontaneous episodic vestibular syndrome (s-EVS)	Brief, spontaneous discrete episodes lasting <24 h then resolving before the next episode
Triggered acute vestibular syndrome (t-AVS)	Triggered by toxins or trauma
Spontaneous acute vestibular syndrome (s-AVS)	Spontaneous episodes lasting >24 h or present at time of examination; does not completely resolve before the next episode
Triggered chronic vestibular syndrome (t-CVS)	Triggered chronic symptoms that do not completely resolve
Spontaneous chronic vestibular syndrome (s-CVS)	Spontaneous chronic symptoms that do not completely resolve

From Newman-Toker DE, Edlow JA. TiTrATE: a novel, evidence-based approach to diagnosing acute dizziness and vertigo. Neurol Clin 2015;33(3):577–99; with permission.

disease processes. The most common causes of t-EVS is BPPV and orthostatic hypotension but mimics include central paroxysmal positional vertigo (CPPV) from posterior fossa mass lesions and intravascular volume loss such as gastrointestinal or retroperitoneal bleed. A thorough history and physical examination using the *Triage-TiTrATE–Test* approach can differentiate between serious and benign pathology (see **Fig. 3**) OR go to infographic: https://connect.johnshopkins.edu/dizzyinfo.

Other Causes of Triggered Episodic Vestibular Syndrome

Other common causes of t-EVS are CPPV, which may be secondary to benign causes such as alcohol intoxication but may also be due to posterior fossa tumor or strokes. Furthermore, CPPV has a specific type of finding, nystagmus, on examination that differentiates it from BPPV. CPPV although is not generally seen without other neurologic findings. (See Video at https://collections.lib.utah.edu/details?id=1213448).[11] Other mimics for vestibular conditions include orthostatic hypotension may be due to benign causes such as dehydration but also from more dangerous causes such as gastrointestinal and retroperitoneal bleeds, myocardial infarct, sepsis, adrenal insufficiency, and diabetic ketoacidosis.

New-Onset Spontaneous Episodic Vestibular Syndrome

A thorough history is required to differentiate causes of s-EVS because most patients are asymptomatic at time of presentation and because no trigger will cause symptoms. Other vestibular mimics include benign disorders such as vestibular migraine, panic attacks, vasovagal syncope, and Meniere disease. Dangerous causes include transient ischemic attack, subarachnoid hemorrhage, arrhythmia, myocardial infarct, unstable angina, pulmonary embolism, hypoglycemia, and carbon monoxide poisoning.[2] Meniere disease typically does not exhibit the entire classic triad of unilateral tinnitus, reversible sensorineural hearing loss, and aural fullness. If a patient presents with low-frequency sensorineural hearing loss with aural symptoms and vertigo attacks, Meniere is probable. However, with new-onset vertigo, hearing loss, and tinnitus presenting to the ED, beware anterior inferior cerebellar artery territory ischemia.[2]

Vestibular migraine diagnosis requires 5 attacks with vestibular symptoms, migraine headache history, and migraine-like symptoms for one-half of the episodes. Duration of symptoms is seconds to days. This is often not associated with headache. Discharge without further testing is acceptable if this is similar to prior episodes with no red flags and low ABCD2 score, otherwise a full transient ischemic attack (TIA) workup should be done.[2]

Neurally mediate syncope is usually associated with lightheadedness and often includes dizziness or vertigo. The diagnosis is suspected based on history and physical examination while ruling out serious causes. The diagnosis is confirmed as an outpatient with a tilt table test.[2]

Central causes of this include TIA and should be suspected in patients with high ABCD2 scores.[2]

Always consider cardiac arrhythmias in patients with unexplained lightheadedness/dizziness without a trigger. A clinician should have a low threshold for a formal echocardiogram and cardiology follow-up.

Acute Vestibular Syndrome

AVS is defined as persistent symptoms for 24 hours, usually lasting days to weeks. Most cases peak after the first week with a slow gradual recovery. The severity of the disease is so powerful that usually patients come to the ED before they have persistent symptoms for full 24 hours; therefore, it is reasonable to group patients with hours of symptoms that still persist at the time of the evaluation and do not abate at rest and have a persistent spontaneous nystagmus. If there is no nystagmus, one cannot reliably differentiate causes of AVS. AVS can be further grouped into disease triggered by a trauma or toxin (t-AVS) or spontaneously (s-AVS).[2]

Traumatic/Toxic Acute Vestibular Syndrome

T-AVS is often a sequelae of blunt head trauma or due to a toxin. Physical examination findings are not reliable because the findings would vary based on the type of trauma that has occurred and the type of toxin that was ingested (**Box 2**).

Types of Trauma in Toxic Acute Vestibular Syndrome

Types of trauma often associated with this disease process include blunt head, blast, whiplash, and barotrauma, which work on direct injury to the vestibular nerve,

---

Box 2
Etiology of triggered acute vestibular syndrome

Trauma
    Barotrauma
    Blast
    Whiplash
    Skull Fracture
    Concussion
    Vertebral Artery Dissection
    Diseases—direct vestibular nerve, labyrinthine concussion, mechanical disruption of inner ear

Toxic
    Aminoglycoside—gait unsteadiness, oscillopsia, carbon monoxide poisoning

labyrinth, or inner ear. Patients may suffer vertebral artery dissection in setting of whiplash. Patient with traumatic brain injuries suffer from postconcussive syndrome, which is a type of t-AVS.

Types of Toxins in Toxic Acute Vestibular Syndrome

Types of toxins that cause t-AVS include alcohol intoxication, anticonvulsant treatment such as phenytoin toxicity, and aminoglycosides such as gentamicin. Gentamicin is usually associated with gait unsteadiness and bouncing vision while walking (oscillopsia). Please see table for list of t-AVS (see **Box 2**).[12]

Spontaneous Acute Vestibular Syndrome

S-AVS is defined as persistent dizziness that last for days to weeks, accompanied by gait instability, nystagmus, and symptoms worsened with head motion. If this is misclassified as episodic vestibular syndrome and if the wrong test is performed, it will worsen the symptoms and induce nausea and vomiting without benefit. Furthermore, an incorrect treatment will be prescribed. The most common cause of s-AVX is acute vestibular neuritis, which is inflammation of the vestibular nerve without hearing loss that is idiopathic and may be due to the Herpes virus.[13] MRI for typical vestibular neuritis is NOT indicated. The treatment is intravenous or oral steroids although evidence of efficacy is limited.[13] Acute vestibular neuritis must be ruled in to rule out an acute cerebellar, brainstem, or inner ear ischemic stroke. A specific physical examination finding called HINTS Plus Hearing (as described in testing section) has been shown to rule in vestibular neuritis. In a patient with AVS, any pattern other than HINTS is central until proved otherwise.

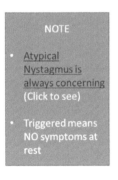

NOTE

- Atypical Nystagmus is always concerning (Click to see)

- Triggered means NO symptoms at rest

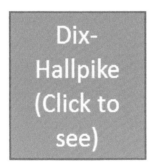

Dix-Hallpike (Click to see)

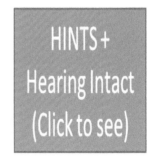

HINTS+ Hearing Intact (Click to see)

TARGETED EXAMINATION + TESTS

Knowledge of typical and atypical nystagmus is a prerequisite in order to correctly diagnose peripheral vertigo and differentiate it from central. Jerk nystagmus is defined as the fast and slow movements of the eye. The direction is defined as the fast direction of the movement. In patients with t-EVS, a Dix-Hallpike will evoke an upbeat torsional nystagmus as shown in **Fig. 4**.

A down beating or ANY spontaneous vertical nystagmus is concerning for a central cause. In AVS, a patient with inflammation of the vestibular nerve called acute vestibular neuritis would be expected to have unidirectional horizontal nystagmus. Direction-changing, gaze-evoked nystagmus (right beating when looking to the right and left beating when looking to the left) in this same setting would be concerning

Nystagmus Types

Upbeat and Torsional Nystagmus with Dix – Hallpike in Episodic Vestibular Syndrome is Posterior Canal BPPV: https://collections.lib.utah.edu/details?id = 1281863

Horizontal Nystagmus that is unidirectional meaning the fast component is in one direction is part of the HINTS diagnosis of Vestibular Neuritis. NOTE: Horizontal Nystagmus can rarely mean central which is why you need all of HINTS to diagnose Peripheral. Horizontal nystagmus is also present in Horizontal Canal BPPV and is direction changing during the exam:
https://collections.lib.utah.edu/details?id = 1277126,
https://collections.lib.utah.edu/details?id = 1281862

Central Paroxsymal Positional Vertigo (CPPV, usually downbeat) and stroke (usually horizontal) can be horizontal direction-changing or vertical direction requires a central process woke up unless it is due to toxins or chronic neurologic condition:
https://collections.lib.utah.edu/details?id = 1295176,
https://collections.lib.utah.edu/details?id = 187733

Down beat torsional rotary is always abnormal and requires w/u for central condition: https://collections.lib.utah.edu/details?id = 1295178

Capture the QR or click on links to see video's from Neurootologist Dr. Dan Gold

Fig. 4. Primer on different nystagmus types.[14–19]

for a central cause. Any other type of nystagmus including torsional and spontaneous vertical is also concerning for a central cause. Central causes may have horizontal nystagmus, which mimics a peripheral cause. Furthermore, visual fixation minimizes peripheral nystagmus; therefore, in order to appreciate a peripheral process visual fixation must be removed using a Penlight test (intermittently shining a light into the patient's eye while watching for nystagmus), Frenzel goggles, or simply placing a sheet of blank paper in front of the patient's field of view during the examination.[20]

Benign Paroxysmal Positional Vertigo

BPPV is the most common form of t-EVS. BPPV is always of brief duration and patients are asymptomatic when not triggered with position changes. Unlike vestibular neuritis, the nystagmus associated with BPPV goes completely away when not triggered. Vestibular neuritis symptoms are still present at rest but worsened with movement. This is an important differentiation because tests such as the Dix-Hallpike will not aide in the diagnosis of vestibular neuritis but will definitely contribute unnecessarily to a patient's feeling of nausea and vomiting. In cases where BPPV is suspected, the clinician should be looking for orthostatic hypotension in patients with positional triggers. Do not misinterpret orthostatic hypotension for orthostatic dizziness. Orthostatic dizziness in the setting of no change in blood pressure may suggest decreased flow to the brain caused by a TIA, cranial vascular stenosis, or intracranial hypotension.[2]

BPPV is caused by calcium carbonate debris that becomes dislodged from the utricle. Calcium carbonate is denser than endolymph; therefore, it will move to the most dependent portions of the canal.[20] The posterior canal is the straightest shot for debris to enter because of its orientation relative to gravity and thus is the cause in 90% of BPPV.[20] [(10)] Particles can enter the horizontal canal and rarely the anterior canal as well, causing different examination findings and requiring different maneuvers to diagnose and treat. Therefore, similar to gallstones or nephrolithiasis, which have a spectrum of disease based on where and how fixed the stone is, these otoliths cause different physical manifestations of dizziness with different gradations of symptoms based on location and their adherence in the canal. The treatment involves moving the otolith from the canal back to the utricle where it came from in all cases, but depending on the location of the otolith certain maneuvers are more effective than others.

Diagnosis and Treatment of Posterior Canal Benign Paroxysmal Positional Vertigo

In the Dix-Hallpike maneuver, the patient is laid down and the affected ear is placed down resulting in an upbeat torsional nystagmus (**Fig. 5**).

If patients cannot tolerate the Dix-Hallpike one can use the side-lying test (**Fig. 6**).

Sometimes the Dix-Hallpike is not positive although they have a great story for BPPV. In cases such as this, consider treatment anyway with close follow-up with a neurologist. The treatment involves using an Epley maneuver as a means of displacing the otolith from the canal back to the utricle (**Fig. 7**).

The treatment for posterior canal BPPV has 90% effectiveness, with a number needed to treat of 1.6.[20] For every 3 patients with posterior canal BPPV, 2 will have complete improvement.[20] BPPV untreated with an Epley has a 46% recurrence risk versus 20%.[6] A percentage of 69.8 had reduced their workload, 63.3% had lost

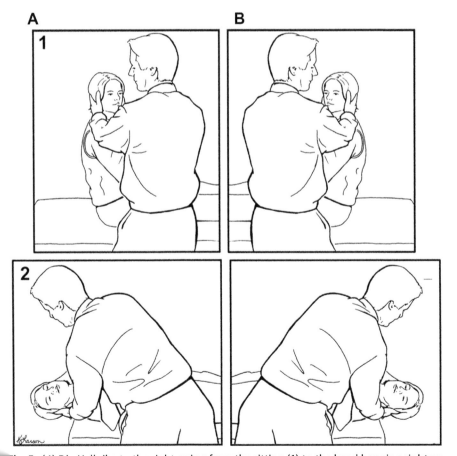

Fig. 5. (*A*) Dix-Hallpike to the right going from the sitting (1) to the head hanging right position (2). (*B*) Dix-Hallpike to the left (see also: https://collections.lib.utah.edu/details?d=177177).[21] (© 2008 Barrow Neurological Institute.)

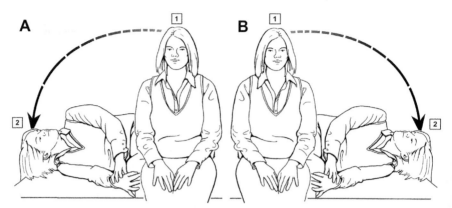

Fig. 6. The side-lying maneuver for posterior canal BPPV on the right (*A*) and left (*B*) sides. (1) The initial upright position; (2) the position to which the patient is moved on each respective side. (© 2008 Barrow Neurological Institute.)

working days, 4.6% had changed their jobs, and 5.7% had quit their jobs due to vertigo symptoms.[7]

Diagnosis and Treatment of Horizontal Canal Benign Positional Vertigo

Horizontal canal benign positional vertigo is much less common based on where the otolith enters. The symptoms can be evoked using the supine roll test (**Fig. 8**).

Lay the patient supine with their head 30° from horizontal. Rotating to the right provokes a horizontal nystagmus beating to the right and rotating to the left has a similar but less intense effect. This is called geotropic horizontal BPPV. There is second type called apogeotropic (which is much less common). Geotropic versus apogeotropic variants are defined by the direction of the horizontal nystagmus and represent different causes in the horizontal canal. The treatment for horizontal canal BPPV is called the Lempert 360 roll maneuver/BBQ roll test (**Fig. 9**).

Horizontal canal BPPV is a self-limited disease process. In fact, there is a technique called forced prolonged positioning, where patients sleeping on the unaffected ear for many hours will also resolve symptoms. About 90% of cases resolve in 1 week and all resolve within 4 weeks.[20]

Although it is worth mentioning that anterior canal BPPV (which is very rare) causes down beat torsional nystagmus, it is important to recognize that if you see this type of nystagmus you must rule out a central cause (see the following stroke mimicking an anterior canal BPPV (https://collections.lib.utah.edu/details?id=1213448)).[11]

The 4 components of HINTS Plus no hearing loss:

- The head impulse test
- Unidirectional gaze-evoked nystagmus
- No skew deviation on eye examination
- Plus no hearing loss

The Head Impulse Test

The head impulse test is often described as positive/abnormal versus negative/normal, which can be confusing. It is much clearer to understand the test by what it is testing. The head impulse test assesses the vestibular-ocular reflex.[22] This reflex has been used for the doll's eye test for coma examination and cold caloric

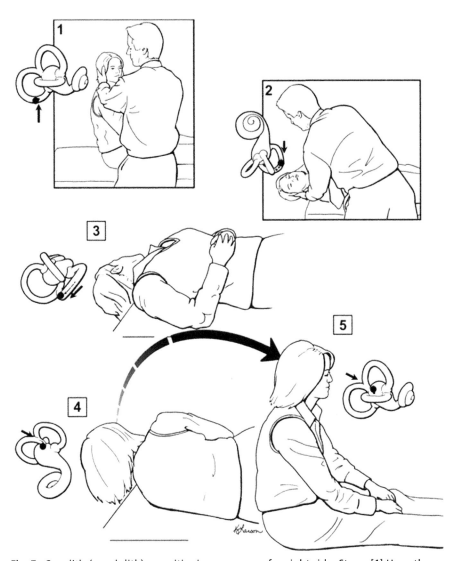

Fig. 7. Canalith (canalolith) repositioning maneuver for right side. Steps: [1] Have the patient sit on a table positioned so that he or she may be laid back to the head-hanging position with the neck in slight extension. Stabilize the head and move it 45° toward the side to be tested. [2] Move the head, neck, and shoulders all together to avoid neck strain. Observe the eyes for nystagmus; hold them open, if necessary. If nystagmus is seen, wait for all nystagmus to abate and hold the position another 15 seconds. [3] While the head is slightly hyperextended, turn the head 90° toward the opposite side and wait 30 seconds. [4] Roll the body to the lateral body position, turn the patient's head toward the ground so that the patient is facing straight down and hold for 15 seconds. [5] While maintaining the head position unchanged relative to the shoulders, have the patient sit up and hold on to the patient for 5 seconds or so to guard against momentary dizziness on sitting up. This maneuver may be repeated several times or until symptoms and nystagmus cannot be reproduced (see https://collections.lib.utah.edu/details?id=1281863).[14] As an alternative, a clinician can use the Semont maneuver; the patient is laid from side to side (see https://collections.lib.utah.edu/details?id=1282656).[23] (© 2008 Barrow Neurological Institute.)

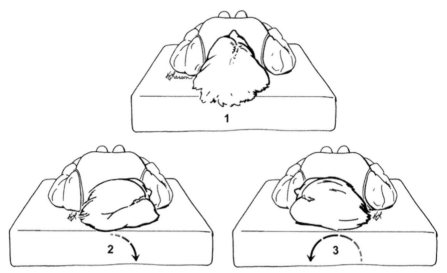

Fig. 8. Supine roll test. The patient's head is moved rapidly from the straight supine position (1) to the right side (2). Observe for horizontal nystagmus and note the direction and intensity. Then move the patient's head back to the straight position (1) for 15 seconds. Then move the head from straight to the head left position (3) and note any nystagmus and its direction and intensity. If the nystagmus is of the geotropic type, the side resulting in the strongest nystagmus is taken to be the affected side (see: https://collections.lib/utah/edu/details?id=177185).[24] (© 2008 Barrow Neurological Institute.)

Lempert Roll Maneuver

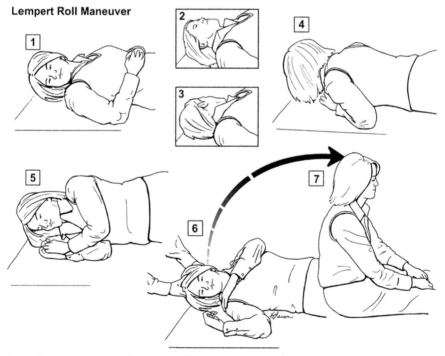

Fig. 9. The Lempert 360 roll maneuver for the treatment of right horizontal canal BPPV with geotropic-type nystagmus. The Lempert 360 roll maneuver for the treatment of right horizontal canal BPPV with geotropic-type nystagmus. Numbers 1 to 7 depict the sequential steps in the maneuver (see https://collections.lib.utah.edu/details?id=187682).[25] (© 2008 Barrow Neurological Institute.)

testing in a comatose patient. When there is inflammation of the vestibular nerve on one side and you turn the head to that side, the reflex that turns the eyes back to center is delayed, causing what is called a corrective "saccade." The head impulse test is a way of moving the head to see that corrective "saccade." Thus a positive test means disruption of the vestibular nerve that is seen in vestibular neuritis. A recent study has shown that emergency physicians perform as well as neuro-otologists when interpreting head impulse testing.[26] The discussion of stroke is found in the neurootology issue of neurology clinics.[8] It there is no corrective "saccade," this is NOT consistent with acute vestibular neuritis and thus requires a central process workup. If there is a catch-up saccade this does not exclusively point to vestibular neuritis and there may still be stroke though and the rest of the HINTS examination must be carried out to rule in the diagnosis and rule out an ischemic stroke (**Fig. 10**).

In acute vestibular neuritis, the patient must experience a horizontal/torsional nystagmus. If no nystagmus is present or if there is vertical or pure torsional component, consider a central cause.[9]

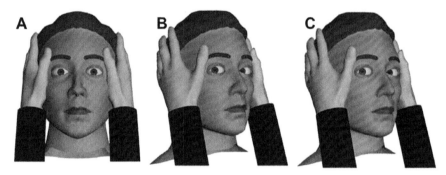

Normal leftward head impulse

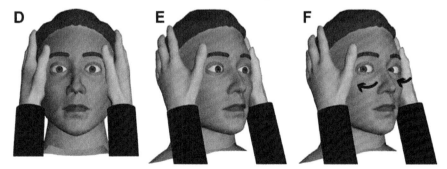

Positive leftward head impulse

Fig. 10. The head impulse test. The top panel illustrates a normal (negative) head impulse test. The subject fixes on a near target (the examiner's nose). (*A*) When the head is turned left, the intact left horizontal vestibuloocular reflex (VOR) produces an equal and opposite eye movement that returns the eye to the target (*B, C*). The bottom panel shows a VOR deficit. (*E*) When the head is turned leftward, the eyes initially move with the head. (*F*) A refixation saccade, or catch-up saccade, returns the eye back to the target (see: https://collections.lib.utah.edu/details?id=177180).[27]

Vertical Skew Deviation

The last step is to look for vertical skew deviation, which is rarely present in vestibular neuritis and points to a central cause.

HINTS has been shown to be more effective at ruling out stroke than MRI and has the reliability to rule in acute vestibular neuritis thus saving on unnecessary tests. Recently it was shown that the addition of hearing loss to HINTS called "HINTS PLUS" even further increased its sensitivity to 99% from 96% (LR+ 32, LR− 0.01) without decreasing its specificity. Please see the following videos to demonstrate the HINTS examination in total[28]: *Demonstration of the steps of HINTS in someone without vertigo:* https://collections.lib.utah.edu/details?id=1209722[29]; *HINTS in vestibular neuritis:* https://collections.lib.utah.edu/details?id=1277126.[30] Patients can be discharged with AVS if they meet the HINTS + No Hearing Loss criteria.

Fig. 2 gives a summary of the treatments of the various peripheral causes of EVS and AVS.

SUMMARY

Dizziness is often a very hard chief complaint to sort out. A systematic approach results in much better differentiation between the likely cause and a life-threatening mimic and allows the clinician to rule out life-threatening causes with better accuracy than a diagnostic study such as an MRI. We are fortunate to have very reliable and accurate physical examination findings in the assessment of the dizzy patient and it presents an opportunity for clinicians to return to the bedside to assess their patients. This technique if used in hands of clinician who has mastered the Triage-TiTraTE-Test approach can result in fewer patients who are incorrectly diagnosed with a benign condition and fewer patients who suffer unnecessarily with a readily treatable disease.

ACKNOWLEDGMENTS

The author would like to acknowledge Dan Gold D.O. for allowing the use of his videos and proofreading this document.

REFERENCES

1. Newman-Toker DE, Hsieh YH, Camargo CA Jr, et al. Spectrum of dizziness visits to US emergency departments: cross-sectional analysis from a nationally representative sample. Mayo Clin Proc 2008;83(7):765–75.
2. Newman-Toker DE, Edlow JA. TiTrATE: a novel, evidence-based approach to diagnosing acute dizziness and vertigo. Neurol Clin 2015;33(3):577–99.
3. Edlow JA. Diagnosing dizziness:we are teaching the wrong paradigm! Acad Emerg Med 2013;20(10):1064–6.
4. Kattah JC, Talkad AV, Wang DZ, et al. HINTS to diagnose stroke in the acute vestibular syndrome: three-step bedside oculomotor examination more sensitive than early MRI diffusion-weighted imaging. Stroke 2009;40(11):3504–10.
5. Kerber KA, Schweigler L, West BT, et al. Value of computed tomography scans in ED dizziness visits: analysis from a nationally representative sample. Am J Emerg Med 2010;28(9):1030–6.
6. Kerber KA, Newman-Toker DE. Misdiagnosing dizzy patients: common pitfalls in clinical practice. Neurol Clin 2015;33(3):565–75.
7. Benecke H, Agus S, Kuessner D, et al. The burden and impact of vertigo: findings from the REVERT patient registry. Front Neurol 2013;4:136.

8. Newman-Toker DE, Kerber KA, Meurer WJ, et al. Emergency neuro-otology: diagnosis and management of acute dizziness and vertigo. Neurol Clin 2015;33(3).
9. Edlow JA. Diagnosing patients with acute-onset persistent dizziness. Ann Emerg Med 2018;71(5):625–31.
10. Spot at end: Newman-Toker DE. A new approach to the dizzy patient PDF. [Neuro-Ophthalmology Virtual Education Library: NOVEL Web Site]. Available at: https://collections.lib.utah.edu/ark:/87278/s6tm7cr7. Accessed October 11, 2018.
11. Gold D. Positional downbeat nystagmus mimicking anterior canal BPPV, [Neuro-Ophthalmology Virtual Education Library: NOVEL Web Site]. Available at: https://collections.lib.utah.edu/details?id=1213448. Accessed October 11, 2018.
12. Fife TD, von Brevern M. Benign paroxysmal positional vertigo in the acute care setting. Neurol Clin 2015;33(3):601–17.
13. Strupp M, Magnusson M. Acute unilateral vestibulopathy. Neurol Clin 2015;33(3): 669–85.
14. Gold D. Posterior canal BPPV pre- and post-Epley maneuver [Neuro-ophthalmology Virtual Education Library: NOVEL]. Available at: https://collections.lib.utah.edu/details?id=1281863. Accessed October 11, 2018.
15. Brune T, Gold D. Vestibular neuritis with + head impulse test and unidirectional nystagmus [Neuro-ophthalmology Virtual Education Library: NOVEL]. Available at: https://collections.lib.utah.edu/ark:/87278/s6546h55. Accessed October 11, 2018.
16. Gold D. The geotropic variant of horizontal canal BPPV, [Neuro-ophthalmology Virtual Education Library: NOVEL]. Available at: https://collections.lib.utah.edu/details?id=1281862. Accessed October 11, 2018.
17. Gold D. Downbeat nystagmus, [Neuro-ophthalmology Virtual Education Library: NOVEL]. Available at: https://collections.lib.utah.edu/details?id=1295176. Accessed October 11, 2018.
18. Gold D. Gaze-evoked and rebound nystagmus in a cerebellar syndrome, [Neuro-ophthalmology Virtual Education Library: NOVEL]. Available at: https://collections.lib.utah.edu/details?id=187733. Accessed October 11, 2018.
19. Gold D. Torsional nystagmus due to medullary pilocytic astrocytoma, [Neuro-ophthalmology Virtual Education Library: NOVEL]. Available at: https://collections.lib.utah.edu/details?id=1295178. Accessed October 11, 2018.
20. Welgampola MS, Bradshaw AP, Lechner C, et al. Bedside assessment of acute dizziness and vertigo. Neurol Clin 2015;33(3):551–64.
21. Newman-Toker D. Dix-Hallpike test for the left posterior semicircular canal [Neuro-ophthalmology Virtual Education Library: NOVEL]. 2018. Available at: https://collections.lib.utah.edu/details?id=177177. Accessed October 11, 2018.
22. Kerber KA. Vertigo and dizziness in the emergency department. Emerg Med Clin North Am 2009;27(1):39–50.
23. Gold D. Posterior canal BPPV treated with Semont maneuver [Neuro-ophthalmology Virtual Education Library: NOVEL]. Available at: https://collections.lib.utah.edu/details?id=1282656. Accessed October 11, 2018.
24. Newman-Toker D. Supine roll test (Pagnini-McClure Maneuver). [Neuro-ophthalmology Virtual Education Library: NOVEL]. Available at: https://collections.lib.utah.edu/details?id=177185. Accessed October 11, 2018.
25. Gold D. Horizontal canal - BPPV: BBQ roll to treat the right side [Neuro-ophthalmology Virtual Education Library: NOVEL]. Available at: https://collections.lib.utah.edu/details?id=187682. Accessed October 11, 2018.

26. Guler A, Karbek Akarca F, Eraslan C, et al. Clinical and video head impulse test in the diagnosis of posterior circulation stroke presenting as acute vestibular syndrome in the emergency department. J Vestib Res 2017;27(4):233–42.
27. Newman-Toker DE. 3-Component H.I.N.T.S. battery [Neuro-ophthalmology Virtual Education Library: NOVEL]. Available at: https://collections.lib.utah.edu/details?id=177180. Accessed October 11, 2018.
28. Newman-Toker DE, Kerber KA, Hsieh YH, et al. HINTS outperforms ABCD2 to screen for stroke in acute continuous vertigo and dizziness. Acad Emerg Med 2013;20(10):986–96.
29. Gold D. Demonstration of HINTS examination in a normal subject. [Neuro-ophthalmology Virtual Education Library: NOVEL]. Available at: https://collections.lib.utah.edu/details?id=1209722. Accessed October 11, 2018.
30. Brune T, Gold D. Vestibular neuritis with + head impulse test and unidirectional nystagmus. [Neuro-ophthalmology Virtual Education Library: NOVEL]. Available at: https://collections.lib.utah.edu/details?id=1277126. Accessed October 11, 2018.

Epistaxis

Neil Alexander Krulewitz, DO*, Megan Leigh Fix, MD

KEYWORDS

• Epistaxis • Anterior epistaxis • Posterior epistaxis • TXA • ENT emergencies

KEY POINTS

• Epistaxis is a common ear, nose, and throat (ENT) emergency and occurs in a bimodal distribution affecting approximately 60% of the population.
• Most epistaxis (90%) arises from an anterior source referred to as Kiesselbach plexus.
• Anterior epistaxis can usually be managed with a combination of topical vasoconstriction, clamping, and cautery. Some cases may require nasal tampons.
• Posterior epistaxis is rare (10%) but should be treated aggressively with posterior packing, ENT consultation, and admission because significant complications can arise.
• There are several simple-to-use and well-tolerated commercial devices to control anterior and posterior epistaxis.
• Tranexamic acid has strong recent evidence for its use in treating epistaxis.

EPIDEMIOLOGY

Epistaxis is a frequently encountered ear, nose, and throat (ENT) condition by emergency providers in the United States, responsible for approximately 1 in 200 emergency department (ED) visits.[1] It is estimated that the lifetime prevalence of epistaxis is approximately 60% within the general population, with about 6% of events resulting in medical treatment.[2–4] Epistaxis most commonly occurs within a bimodal age distribution, primarily affecting individuals aged 2 to 10 years and aged 50 to 80 years.[4] Peak incidence occurs among those aged 70 years and older, with this patient group 3 times more likely to seek medical care than pediatric patients.[1] Although rarely a direct cause of mortality, epistaxis may induce significant morbidity, particularly in the elderly and those with coexisting cardiovascular disease. This condition often presents management challenges for emergency providers.[5]

ANATOMY

The nose is richly vascularized. This vascular supply is composed of multiple anastomoses that originate from branches of both the internal and external carotid arteries.

Disclosure Statement: The authors have no disclosures.
Division of Emergency Medicine, University of Utah, 30 North 1900 East, Room 1C26, Salt Lake City, UT 84132, USA
* Corresponding author.
E-mail address: Neil.Krulewitz@hsc.utah.edu

Emerg Med Clin N Am 37 (2019) 29–39
https://doi.org/10.1016/j.emc.2018.09.005
0733-8627/19/© 2018 Elsevier Inc. All rights reserved.
emed.theclinics.com

The anterior nasal septum receives its vascular supply from the anterior and posterior ethmoidal arteries, branches of the internal carotid artery, which enter the nasal cavity superiorly. Additionally, contributions are made from branches of the internal maxillary artery, including the sphenopalatine artery (SPA) posteriorly and the greater palatine artery inferiorly, as well as the superior labial artery, a branch of the facial artery.[6] The anastomosis of these various vessels is commonly referred to as Kiesselbach plexus, which is the most common site of anterior epistaxis. The posterior nasal septum and the lateral nasal wall (inferior to the middle turbinates) receive vascular supply from the SPA and terminal branches of the maxillary artery.[3] Posterior epistaxis is generally attributable to bleeding from these sources (**Fig. 1**).

CLASSIFICATION

Clinically, epistaxis is most often classified as either anterior or posterior, which is determined by the anatomic source of bleeding. Approximately 80% to 90% of epistaxis occurs along the anterior nasal septum, most of which arise from Kiesselbach plexus.[7] Anterior sources of bleeding are generally less challenging for the emergency provider to treat because most involve smaller vessels and are more readily compressible and amenable to electrocautery and topical treatment.[8] In contrast, approximately 10% of epistaxis episodes are attributable to a posterior source.[3,4] Posterior epistaxis is often significantly more difficult to identify and manage, is commonly arterial in origin, and presents a greater risk of aspiration and challenge in achieving hemostasis.

Epistaxis may be further classified as primary or secondary. Primary causes of epistaxis are often idiopathic and arise spontaneously without any obvious precipitating insult, although environmental factors likely contribute (see later discussion). Primary epistaxis accounts for approximately 85% of all events.[4,9] Epistaxis may also be secondary to an identifiable cause, including trauma, postsurgical, vascular abnormalities, inherited or acquired coagulopathies, and anticoagulant use, among others.

ETIOLOGIC FACTORS

There are numerous factors that may precipitate epistaxis, many of which can be subdivided into groups (see later discussion) and are reviewed in **Box 1**. In most cases, the cause of epistaxis remains idiopathic.[4] Regardless of age or other risk factors,

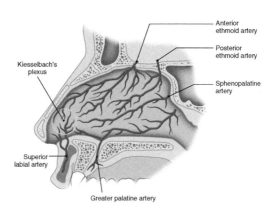

Fig. 1. Anatomy of the blood supply to the nose. (*Courtesy of* Christy Krames, Austin, TX.)

Box 1
Etiologic factors of epistaxis

- Trauma
  - Digital trauma
  - Facial trauma
  - Foreign body insertion
  - Septal perforation
  - Barotrauma
  - Illicit drug use

- Metabolic
  - Hepatic dysfunction
  - Renal failure
  - Uremia
  - Alcohol

- Autoimmune
  - Hemophilia
  - Leukemia
  - von Willebrand disease

- Vascular abnormality
  - Hereditary hemorrhagic telangiectasia
  - Congestive heart failure
  - Hypertension
  - Diabetes
  - Granulomatosis with polyangiitis (formerly Wegener granulomatosis)

- Iatrogenic
  - Anticoagulation (warfarin, new oral anticoagulant drugs)
  - Antiplatelet agents (aspirin, clopidogrel)
  - Nonsteroidal antiinflammatory drugs
  - Intranasal medications
  - Postsurgical
  - Direct trauma (passage of tubes, nasotracheal intubation, nasogastric tubes)

- Idiopathic

- Neoplastic
  - Juvenile angiofibroma
  - Nasopharyngeal carcinoma
  - Squamous cell cancer
  - Paranasal sinus tumor

- Inflammatory
  - Rhinosinusitis
  - Nasal polyps
  - Nasal diphtheria

- Congenital
  - Septal deviation
  - Septal spur

---

patients are significantly more likely to experience epistaxis during the winter months in colder climates. This is likely attributable to decreased temperatures and exposure to indoor heating during this period, which result in low ambient humidity and increased evaporation of water from nasal mucosa, predisposing to desiccation and epistaxis.[10]

Local trauma to the nasal mucosa is a common precipitant of epistaxis, responsible for approximately 17% of epistaxis visits to the ED[1] and the most common cause of epistaxis among the pediatric population.[11] Children may often present with epistaxis after digital trauma or local irritation from foreign bodies. Other sources of local trauma can induce epistaxis, including nasal or facial bone fractures, foreign body insertion, septal perforation from substance abuse, iatrogenic manipulation, and neoplasm.

Numerous systemic conditions can also predispose to epistaxis. Inherited bleeding diatheses, including hemophilia and von Willebrand disease, as well as acquired coagulopathies, often secondary to medications or liver disease, may cause initial or recurrent epistaxis.[12,13] Recent literature suggests that elevated nasal venous pressures can predispose to epistaxis.[13] Hypertension and diabetes are minor risk factors for recurrent epistaxis, possibly due to atherosclerotic changes in the vasculature resulting in increased venous pressure the nasal vessels.[13] However, there exists a high association between congestive heart failure (CHF) and recurrent epistaxis, again related to elevated nasal venous pressures, rather than bleeding from Kiesselbach plexus.[13,14] Additionally, hereditary hemorrhagic telangiectasia often manifests with nasal mucosal telangiectasias, presenting frequently with recurrent epistaxis that is often refractory to standard techniques.[15,16]

An ongoing debate in the literature exists regarding the association between hypertension and epistaxis; however, a causal relationship between the two has yet to be established. Is it proposed that hypertension is seldom the direct cause of epistaxis but is rather related to underlying vascular disease or associated with anxiety during an episode of epistaxis.[9] Given the absence of evidence demonstrating a causal relationship, and per the American College of Emergency Physicians recommendations, acute epistaxis therapies should be directed toward control of bleeding, rather than reduction of blood pressure.[17]

PATIENT HISTORY

Initial evaluation of the patient presenting with epistaxis necessitates first assessing the patient's airway, breathing, and circulation (ABC). Evidence of clinical instability, including tachycardia, hypotension, airway compromise, respiratory distress, or altered mental status, requires prompt intervention. Hemodynamic stabilization and airway management are paramount and should take priority over cessation of epistaxis in this setting (see later discussion).

In the individual with epistaxis who is hemodynamically stable and not in respiratory distress, obtaining a thorough patient history can be exceptionally helpful in establishing an underlying cause, and may direct further workup and definitive management of the bleeding. Important factors to consider in the history include onset, duration of symptoms, laterality and quantity of bleeding, and any preceding trauma.[18] Patients with posterior epistaxis may experience bleeding from bilateral nares, a large volume of blood in the posterior oropharynx, and hematemesis or hemoptysis.[4,17] If the patient has suffered from prior episodes of epistaxis, it may be helpful to elucidate prior interventions that have been successful in achieving hemostasis.

Frequent episodes of epistaxis may indicate an underlying pathologic condition contributing to recurrent bleeding. A targeted past medical history should be obtained and may provide evidence to suggest an underlying disorder. Consideration should be given to history of cirrhosis or hepatic impairment, renal insufficiency, malignancy, hypertension, and CHF, as well as hereditary coagulopathies or anatomic abnormalities that may predispose to the development of epistaxis. Additionally, a review of systems may include the presence of skin rash (petechiae or purpura), frequent easy bruising, melena, and hematochezia,[4,17] which may indicate underlying coagulopathy and provide insight into the severity of bleeding. It is equally vital to review the patient's medications because use of anticoagulants, antiplatelet agents (eg, aspirin and tica-grelor), and nonsteroidal antiinflammatory drugs may predispose to the development of epistaxis and require additional interventions to achieve hemostasis.[4,13]

Social history, including drug and alcohol use, as well as smoking, should not be overlooked. The use of intranasal cocaine or other drugs of abuse should be addressed with the patient.

MANAGEMENT
Resuscitation

Although rarely-life threatening, epistaxis requires an initial evaluation focused on the patient's ABC. Hemodynamic stability must be assessed expeditiously by monitoring vital signs and clinical appearance because large-volume epistaxis may induce signif-icant morbidity in patients with existing comorbidities and concomitant cardiovascular disease. Large-bore intravenous access for fluid resuscitation should be obtained early in unstable patients, and a rapid assessment made to ensure that the patient does not require emergent airway management.[7,19]

A complete blood count may be obtained to assess for degree of hemorrhage. A complete metabolic panel should be ordered to evaluate for renal or hepatic dysfunc-tion, as well as the breakdown products of large quantities of ingested blood.[19] If large-volume hemorrhage is suspected, a type and screen or a type and cross should be performed, as appropriate. Routine coagulation profiles, including prothrombin time or international normalized ratio and partial thromboplastin time are not recommended unless the patient has a known coagulopathy, takes anticoagulation medications, is a pediatric patient, or the provider has a high clinical suspicion for a bleeding diathesis based on history and presentation.[19,20] Patients with coagulopathies may require emergent correction with specific anticoagulation reversal agents, vitamin K, fresh frozen plasma, prothrombin complex concentrate, or other appropriate intervention.

Assessment

If the patient is experiencing active bleeding, encourage the patient to lean forward to reduce swallowing or aspiration of blood. Instruct the patient to apply direct pressure to the cartilaginous portion of the nose just below the nasal bones to attempt to tam-ponade bleeding. For optimal, unobstructed visualization of the nasal mucosa, it is recommended to instruct the patient to blow their nose into a tissue to clear any exist-ing clot, followed by administration of a topical vasoconstrictor and application of direct pressure to the nasal mucosa for a minimum of 15 minutes.[19,21] Use of nasal clips for the purpose of achieving hemostasis has been demonstrated to be signifi-cantly more efficacious than manual nasal compression.[21] A vasoconstrictor, typically an alpha-agonist, such as oxymetazoline (Afrin), may be applied via topical spray. Alternatively, cotton balls may be soaked with the vasoconstrictor and inserted into the nasal cavity.[4] This method reduces hemorrhage after the clot has been cleared to enable better visualization of the nasal mucosa. If the patient is having significant discomfort, a topical anesthetic may also be applied. Frequently used topical vaso-constrictors and anesthetics, and recommended equipment for epistaxis are listed in **Boxes 2** and **3**, respectively.

To thoroughly examine the patient's nasal cavity, proper preparation and setup are critical. The examiner should have the bed positioned at the appropriate height and gloves, face mask, eye protection, suction, and nasal speculum should be available. Using a headlamp for the light source is ideal because this enables the examiner to use both hands freely. With the nasal speculum, carefully examine the anterior nasal

---

Box 2
Recommended topical medications

Topical vasoconstrictors[19]

- 0.05% oxymetazoline (Afrin)
- 0.5% phenylephrine hydrochloride
- 1:1000 epinephrine
- 4% cocaine

Topical anesthetics[22]

- 4% lidocaine, 0.1% epinephrine, 0.4% tetracaine (LET) solution
- 4% lidocaine

Data from Barnes ML, Spielmann PM, White PS. Epistaxis: a contemporary evidence based approach. Otolaryngol Clin North Am 2012;45:1005–17; and Simon E. The emergency department management of posterior epistaxis. 2016. Available at: http://www.emdocs.net/emergency-department-management-posterior-epistaxis/. Accessed October, 2017.

---

septum and lateral walls, closely noting the Little area for any evidence of bleeding or scabbed or dry areas.

Inability to visualize an anterior source of bleeding, bilateral bleeding from the nares, or significant blood in the posterior oropharynx all suggest a posterior source of epistaxis (see later discussion of management of this scenario).

Anterior Epistaxis

If an anterior source of bleeding is identified, definitive management should proceed. If administration of topical vasoconstrictors and direct compression alone fail to achieve adequate hemostasis, and an anterior source has been identified, cautery is the next

---

Box 3
Recommended equipment for epistaxis

- Head lamp or light source
- Nasal clamp
- Tissues
- Cotton balls
- Suction
- Nasal speculum
- Bayonet forceps
- Topical vasoconstrictor or anesthetics
- Silver nitrate sticks
- Prepackaged nasal tampon or balloons
- TXA
- Surgicel or gelfoam
- Foley catheters (for posterior epistaxis)
- Prepackaged long tampon or double balloon (posterior epistaxis)

---

recommended step in control of epistaxis.[3,8,19] Cautery, either electrical or via silver nitrate, is associated with greater rates of treatment success and lower pain scores than anterior nasal packing.[8,23] Silver nitrate cautery should be performed by touching the dry salt silver nitrate–tipped applicator to moist mucosa, with the objective of direct cautery of the bleeding site. It may be beneficial, however, to initially cauterize circumferentially around the bleeding site to better control hemorrhage.[3,19] Cautery must be performed with caution to avoid nasal septal perforation, with application to only a small area and for a short duration of time. It should never be performed bilaterally, which increases risk of septal perforation.[19]

If cautery fails to achieve adequate hemostasis, or bleeding is too excessive to properly visualize or perform cautery, anterior nasal packing has often been the standard next approach in treatment. Recent literature suggests that before proceeding to anterior nasal packing, tranexamic acid (TXA) may be a preferable, alternative next step in achieving hemostasis.[8,24] TXA is an antifibrinolytic agent used in a variety of settings to reduce hemorrhage. In a randomized controlled trial, anterior packing with TXA-soaked cotton pledgets (500 mg in 5 mL of injectable TXA) was compared with packing with standard therapy (cotton pledgets soaked in 1:100,000 epinephrine and 2% lidocaine). TXA pledgets were removed with cessation of bleeding, whereas standard packing was removed after 3 days. This study found that bleeding cessation occurred within 10 minutes in 71% of subjects in the TXA group, whereas only 31% of the standard group achieved hemostasis in this period.[24] Additionally, a significantly larger number of subjects who received TXA treatment were discharged from the ED within 2 hours compared with the group receiving standard therapy (95.3% vs 6.4%), resulting in much higher patient satisfaction.[24] Although further study is necessary, it may be reasonable to consider using TXA for control of anterior epistaxis refractory to cautery and before proceeding with anterior packing.

If local therapy and cauterization fail to control bleeding, the provider should attempt to control hemorrhage with nasal packing. At this point in the evaluation, the provider should strongly consider if this may be a posterior bleed, noting examination findings mentioned previously. If anterior epistaxis is still suspected, there are several modern, commercial products available that are relatively easily inserted by emergency providers. Nasal packing works by applying direct pressure to the anterior nasal mucosa, with the objective of tamponading the bleed (**Fig. 2**).

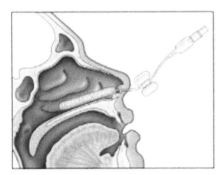

Insert nasal tampon along superior aspect of hard palate

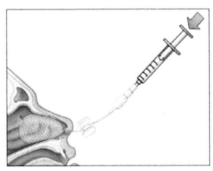

Follow specific product directions to inflate the balloon to tamponade bleeding in the anterior nares

Fig. 2. Insertion of a modern commercial nasal tampon. (*Courtesy of* Smith & Nephew, © 2018.)

Although traditional nasal packing often involved layering lubricated or antibiotic-soaked gauze into the nasal cavity, this has generally fallen out of favor for more simple-to-use commercial products. The nasal tampon is typically first-line for uncomplicated anterior nasal bleeding. Multiple products, including polyvinyl acetyl polymer sponges, Merocel (Medtronic, Minneapolis, MN, USA), and inflatable nasal balloons, Rapid Rhino (AnthroCare Corp, Austin, TX, USA) are available to pack the anterior nasal cavity.[3,4,19] The Rapid Rhino is additionally reported to include a procoagulant outer surface that acts as a platelet aggregator, which may aid in hemostasis in patients on antiplatelet and anticoagulant therapy.[4,19] The Rapid Rhino should be submerged in sterile water for 30 seconds before its insertion along the septal floor, parallel to the hard palate, and then a 20 mL syringe is used to inflate the balloon until the pilot cuff is firm.[17] It is recommended that anterior nasal packs are lubricated with petroleum jelly or antibiotic ointment on insertion. This will aid in insertion and help to prevent occurrence of potentially fatal toxic-shock syndrome by release of exotoxins by Staphylococcus aureus bacteria.[3] Bayonet forceps may aid in the insertion of nasal tampons. Packing is generally left in place for a minimum of 24 hours. Patients with multiple comorbidities or severe hemorrhage may warrant admission for observation and antibiotic administration, particularly if bilateral packing is necessary to achieve hemostasis.[19] A 2015 study in the Annals of Emergency Medicine by Cohn[25] reviewed the recent literature addressing the administration of prophylactic antibiotics for patients undergoing nasal packing and found no increased incidence of local infection, sinusitis, or toxic shock syndrome in patients with packing in place for 24 to 48 hours. Given increased risk of complications associated with antibiotic administration, including Clostridium difficile and Stevens-Johnson syndrome, it may be reasonable to withhold antibiotics in low-risk patients in whom packing will be removed within 48 hours. Antibiotics should still be strongly considered, however, in patients who are immunocompromised, have valvular heart disease, or those receiving posterior packing.[17,25] It is also reasonable to defer this decision to the consulting ENT physician who will be following the patient.

Anterior nasal packing is often associated with significant discomfort for the patient and may cause long-term side effects.[23] Long-term pain was described in 8% of individuals who underwent cautery, whereas 26% of subjects who received nasal packing reported significant pain. Common side effects of nasal packing include nasal crusting and impaired breathing.[23]

In patients in whom good hemostasis is achieved without nasal packing, a topical ointment, such as paraffin, chlorhexidine or phenylephrine (Nasalate), or triamcinolone should be prescribed for 7 days to moisturize the nasal mucosa and reduce the risk of rebleeding.[4] Patients should be educated about proper nasal clamping technique and should have regular follow-up with their primary care physicians.

Posterior Epistaxis

Posterior epistaxis is almost always limited to adult patients because children usually suffer from anterior bleeds secondary to digital trauma or foreign bodies.[22] As mentioned previously, posterior epistaxis should be considered if there is inability to visualize an anterior source of bleeding or if there is bilateral bleeding. Additional evidence to suggest posterior epistaxis includes symptoms of nausea, hematemesis, and hemoptysis. Additionally, if anterior bleeding is suspected and treated with an anterior pack but there is continued bleeding around the pack or visualization of bleeding in the posterior oropharynx despite the anterior pack, posterior bleed should be suspected.

The initial approach for posterior epistaxis is similar to what is described previously for anterior epistaxis. If a posterior source is suspected or anterior management does not control bleeding, then posterior epistaxis management should ensue. This necessitates a type of posterior pack, which can be accomplished with a Foley catheter, nasal tampon, or an inflatable nasal balloon catheter. It should be noted that studies have concluded that posterior packing is very painful, and procedural sedation and/or narcotic pain control should be considered when appropriate.[26] In addition, all posterior epistaxis should be managed in consultation with an ENT specialist.

The Foley catheter is cited as the most commonly used posterior nasal packing device.[22] In this technique, a lubricated catheter (size 10F, 12F, or 14F) is advanced into the nasopharynx and then partially inflated with approximately 5 to 10 mL of saline. Traction is applied until the balloon is seated against the posterior choana to tamponade bleeding. The Foley catheter is then clamped in place using an umbilical clamp. After placing the Foley, an anterior pack should also placed in the affected naris. It is critical to apply padding with gauze to protect the soft tissues of the nose and prevent soft tissue necrosis.

As with anterior epistaxis, there are also multiple commercially available posterior nasal packing devices, including Rapid Rhino, Epi-Max (Boston Medical Products, Shrewsbury, MA, USA), and T3100 Epistaxis Catheter (Bausch & Lomb, Rochester, NY, USA).[3,22,26] Typically, these products have 2 balloons: 1 anterior and 1 posterior. After proper pain control, positioning, and topical anesthesia, the device is inserted. Then the posterior balloon is inflated and withdrawn forward until the posterior balloon is seated. Then the anterior balloon is inflated to tamponade the anterior nasal cavity. These devices should be pretreated with antibiotic ointment to aid insertion and help prevent toxic-shock syndrome.[22,26]

It is recommended that all patients with posterior nasal packing be admitted for observation and receive systemic antibiotics.[4,17,22,26] Serious complications, such as arrhythmia and death, have been described; however, these are rare.[27] Other complications include bradycardia and hypotension from increased vagal tone,

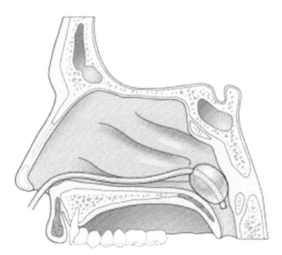

Fig. 3. Foley catheter insertion in epistaxis. Note the tip of the catheter in the posterior oropharynx. At this point the catheter may be inflated and the opposite end withdrawn to tamponade posterior bleeding. (*Reprinted from* Maxillofacial trauma and esthetic facial reconstruction. 2nd edition. In: Eppley BL, editor. Primary repair of facial soft tissue injuries. p. 342–67. Copyright 2012; with permission from Elsevier.)

hypoventilation, hypoxia, aspiration, syncope, nasal septal necrosis, and toxic shock syndrome. Most recommendations on antibiotics include cephalexin, amoxicillin or clavulanic acid, or trimethoprim-sulfamethoxazole.[17,22] Packing should generally be removed in approximately 72 hours in conjunction with ENT consultation.[22,26,27] Patients with posterior epistaxis that is not controlled by the above-mentioned methods will need surgical intervention by an ENT provider, including endoscopic evaluation and potentially ligation or embolization[4,22] (**Fig. 3**).

SUMMARY AND RECOMMENDATIONS

Epistaxis is a common ENT emergency encountered by emergency providers. Although there are no large randomized controlled trials to recommend an approach, the authors' recommendations are as follows.

After stabilizing the patient's ABC, perform a thorough history and physical examination to elucidate the cause and source of bleeding. If an anterior bleed is suspected, instruct the patient to blow the nose to eliminate clot, and apply a topical vasoconstrictor and/or anesthetic and clamp the nares for at least 15 minutes. If this has failed to control the bleeding and an anterior source has been identified, cautery with silver nitrate can be attempted. If this is unsuccessful, consider TXA-soaked cotton pledgets and then proceed to a commercially available anterior nasal tampon. If posterior bleed is suspected, pain control and procedural sedation should be considered, followed by either insertion of a Foley catheter and subsequent anterior pack or a commercially available dual balloon posterior packing device. If bleeding continues after anterior packing or in the setting of a posterior bleed, ENT consultation is advised.

REFERENCES

1. Pallin DJ, Chng YM, McKay MP, et al. Epidemiology of epistaxis in US emergency departments, 1992 to 2001. Ann Emerg Med 2005;46:77–81.
2. Tomkinson A, Roblin DG, Flanagan P, et al. Patterns of hospital attendance with epistaxis. Rhinology 1997;35:129–31.
3. Viehweg TL, Roberson JB, Hudson JW. Epistaxis: diagnosis and treatment. J Oral Maxillofac Surg 2006;64:511–8.
4. Yau S. An update on epistaxis. Aust Fam Physician 2015;44:653–6.
5. Bleach NR, Williamson PA, Mady SM. Emergency workload in otolaryngology. Ann R Coll Surg Engl 1994;76:335–8.
6. Koh E, Frazzini V, Kagetsu NJ. Epistaxis: vascular anatomy, origins, and endovascular treatment. AJR Am J Roentgenol 2000;174:845–51.
7. Schlosser RJ. Clinical practice: epistaxis. N Engl J Med 2009;360:784–9.
8. Logan JK, Pantle H. Role of topical tranexamic acid in the management of idiopathic anterior epistaxis in adult patients in the emergency department. Am J Health Syst Pharm 2016;73:1755–9.
9. Melia L, McGarry GW. Epistaxis: update on management. Curr Opin Otolaryngol Head Neck Surg 2011;19:30–5.
10. Purkey MR, Seeskin Z, Chandra R. Seasonal variation and predictors of epistaxis. Laryngoscope 2014;124:2028–33.
11. Gilyoma J, Chalya P. Etiological profile and treatment outcome of epistaxis at a tertiary care hospital in Northwestern Tanzania: a prospective review of 104 cases. BMC Ear Nose Throat Disord 2011;11:8.
12. Middleton P. Epistaxis. Emerg Med Australas 2004;16:428–40.

13. Abrich V, Brozek A, Boyle T, et al. Risk factors for recurrent spontaneous epistaxis. Mayo Clin Proc 2014;89:1636–43.
14. Kanowitz SJ, Citardi MJ, Batra PS. Contemporary management strategies for epistaxis. In: Stucker FS, De Souza C, Lian TS, et al, editors. Rhinology and facial plastic surgery. Leipzig (Germany): Springer; 2009. p. 139–48.
15. Parambil J, Woodard T, Koc O. Pazopanib effective for bevacizumab-unresponsive epistaxis in hereditary hemorrhagic telangiectasia. Laryngoscope 2018. [Epub ahead of print].
16. Halderman A, Ryan M, Clark C, et al. Medical treatment of epistaxis in hereditary hemorrhagic telangiectasia: an evidence-based review. Int Forum Allergy Rhinol 2018;8:729–36.
17. Gilman C. Treatment of epistaxis. 2009. Available at: http://www.acepnow.com/article/treatment-epistaxis/?singlepage=1&theme=print-friendly. Accessed November 2017.
18. Nguyen A. Epistaxis. 2011. Available at: http://emedicine.medscape.com/article/863320-overview. Accessed October 2017.
19. Barnes ML, Spielmann PM, White PS. Epistaxis: a contemporary evidence based approach. Otolaryngol Clin North Am 2012;45:1005–17.
20. Hodgson D, Burdett-Smith P. BET 2: routine coagulation testing in adult patients with epistaxis. Emerg Med J 2011;28:633–4.
21. Hajimaghsoudi M, Largani HA, Baradaranfar MH, et al. A novel method for epistaxis management: randomized clinical trial comparing nose clip with manual compression. Am J Emerg Med 2018;36:149–50.
22. Simon E. The emergency department management of posterior epistaxis. 2016. Available at: http://www.emdocs.net/emergency-department-management-posterior-epistaxis/. Accessed October 2017.
23. Kindler RM, Holzmann D, Landis BN, et al. The high rate of long-term recurrences and sequelae after epistaxis treatment. Auris Nasus Larynx 2016;43:412–7.
24. Zahed R, Moharamzadeh P, Alizadeharasi S, et al. A new and rapid method for epistaxis treatment using injectable form of tranexamic acid topically : a randomized controlled trial. Am J Emerg Med 2013;3:1389–92.
25. Cohn B. Are prophylactic antibiotics necessary for anterior nasal packing in epistaxis? Ann Emerg Med 2015;65:109–11.
26. Goralnick E. Posterior epistaxis nasal pack. 2016. Available at: http://emedicine.medscape.com/article/80545-overview#a1. Accessed May 2018.
27. Monte E, Belmont M, Wax M. Management paradigms for posterior epistaxis: a comparison of costs and complications. Otolaryngol Head Neck Surg 1999;121:103–6.

Sinusitis Update

Benjamin Wyler, MD, MPH, DTMH[a],*, William K. Mallon, MD, DTMH[b]

KEYWORDS

- Sinusitis • Rhinosinusitis • Diagnostic criteria • Antibiotics • Complications
- Sinus imaging

KEY POINTS

- Rhinosinusitis is a common clinical problem in both pediatric and adult patients.
- Rhinosinusitis is usually viral or allergic and does not require antibiotics or imaging of any kind.
- Antibiotics (amoxicillin is first line) should be reserved for patients meeting strict diagnostic criteria for bacterial rhinosinusitis.
- Emergency physicians must also recognize the atypical and complicated cases in which rhinosinusitis causes both morbidity and mortality.

INTRODUCTION

Rhinosinusitis is a common illness in the United States, accounting for more than 3 million ambulatory care visits per year and affecting approximately 1 in 6 adults annually. Total direct health care expenditures associated with these patients are estimated at $3.4 billion annually, a large component of which is medication costs. In addition, there are significant costs associated with lost work and diminished productivity.[1,2] Unnecessary imaging further adds to the overall costs. Rhinosinusitis involves inflammation or infection of the sinus mucosa, which is continuous with the mucosa of the nasopharynx. Therefore, the microbiology of sinusitis overlaps with rhinitis, pharyngitis, and otitis media.

Rhinosinusitis comprises a heterogeneous group of related conditions, and can be categorized based on anatomic location, duration of symptoms, and infectious, allergic, or inflammatory etiology. Most cases of acute sinusitis are due to viral pathogens, and thus do not require antibiotics. Clinical, laboratory, and imaging findings correlate relatively poorly with the gold standard of diagnosis: antral puncture and

Author Disclosures: Neither author has any disclosures, or any conflicts of interest.
[a] Department of Emergency Medicine, Stony Brook University (SUNY), 101 Nicholls Road, HSC Level 4, Stony Brook, NY 11794, USA; [b] Department of Emergency Medicine, Division of International EM Stony Brook University (SUNY), 101 Nicholls Road, HSC Level 4, Stony Brook, NY 11794, USA
* Corresponding author. 19 Spring Hollow Road, Saint James, NY 11780.
E-mail address: bwyler@gmail.com

Emerg Med Clin N Am 37 (2019) 41–54
https://doi.org/10.1016/j.emc.2018.09.007
0733-8627/19/© 2018 Elsevier Inc. All rights reserved.
emed.theclinics.com

mucus aspirate culture, which is rarely performed. Approximately two-thirds of patients have significant improvement in the absence of treatment, and there is only modest benefit from any treatment, including antibiotics and steroids.

Complications of rhinosinusitis are uncommon but can be life threatening and difficult to recognize in the early stages. They include intracranial abscess, orbital cellulitis or abscess, meningitis, osteomyelitis, and septic cavernous sinus thrombosis (CST). Recognition of rare complications is an important element of emergency department diagnosis and treatment.

ANATOMY

The paranasal sinuses comprise four pairs of air-filled cavities surrounding and in continuity with the nasal cavity. The sinuses are named based on the skull bones from which they derive: frontal, maxillary, ethmoid, and sphenoid. They can generally be thought of in relation to the orbits as being superior, inferior, medial, and posterior, respectively.

The sinuses form via the excavation of bone by pneumatic diverticula derived from the nasal cavity and are lined by mucoperiosteum. The maxillary sinus is the first to pneumatize, followed by the ethmoid and frontal sinuses. All sinuses are well pneumatized by age 12 years.

The maxillary sinus contains the infraorbital nerve, and its posteromedial wall abuts the pterygopalatine fossa, which contains the maxillary artery and nerve. The thin alveolar process separates the maxillary sinus from the roots of canine and molar teeth (**Fig. 1**). The ethmoid sinus' lateral margin is the lamina papyracea, a very thin bone forming the medial wall of the orbit. The sphenoid sinuses are located adjacent to the optic canals, dura mater, cavernous sinuses, cranial nerves III to VI, and the internal carotid arteries (**Fig. 2**).

Ostia of the sinuses are important for drainage of sinus secretions. The ostiomeatal complex is a common channel that links the frontal sinus, anterior ethmoid air cells, and the maxillary sinus to the middle meatus, allowing for mucociliary drainage (**Fig. 3**). Occlusion of this critical channel will lead to pansinusitis.

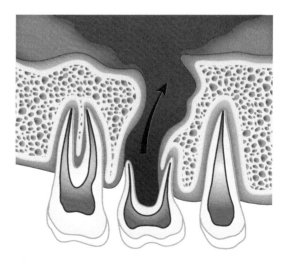

Fig. 1. Apical alveolar abscess erodes through floor of maxillary sinus.

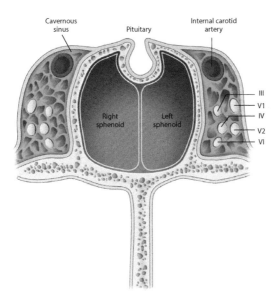

Fig. 2. Sphenoid sinuses and important adjacent neurovascular structures.

CLINICAL FEATURES AND DEFINITIONS

Sinusitis occurs when the mucosal lining of the paranasal sinuses becomes inflamed. Because this mucosa is contiguous with the mucosa of the nasal passages, the two are often concurrently affected, and the condition is referred to as "rhinosinusitis." The pathophysiology of rhinosinusitis includes mucosal edema, sinus ostia obstruction, and ciliary dysfunction.

Sinusitis causes a constellation of symptoms, including nasal congestion or obstruction, nasal discharge, postnasal drip, facial pain, altered sense of smell, fever, headache, dental pain, and halitosis. Symptoms of acute bacterial rhinosinusitis (ABRS) and uncomplicated viral upper respiratory infection (URI) overlap considerably, and it is symptom persistence without improvement that suggests a diagnosis of ABRS.[3] Allergy, local irritants, and barotrauma can also produce similar symptoms.[4] Most barotrauma cases are due to unequalized pressures during descent, and may involve epistaxis.[5]

Sinusitis is classified as acute, subacute, chronic, or recurrent based on the duration and frequency of symptoms (**Table 1**).[3,4,6] Several special circumstances, disease states, and chronic conditions are relevant to rhinosinusitis and should be identified (**Table 2**). These include cystic fibrosis, asthma, immunocompromise, nasal polyps, allergies, and ciliary dyskinesis.[7]

DIAGNOSIS

Diagnosis of ABRS overlaps significantly with viral URI with similar physical examination findings, such as nasal turbinate edema and erythema and sinus percussion tenderness. Transillumination, laboratory testing, sinus imaging, and culture results are of limited utility.[3]

Clinical Diagnostic Criteria

A useful mnemonic to aid in the clinical identification of sinusitis is PODS: facial *P*ain, *P*ressure, or fullness; nasal *O*bstruction; nasal purulence or discolored postnasal

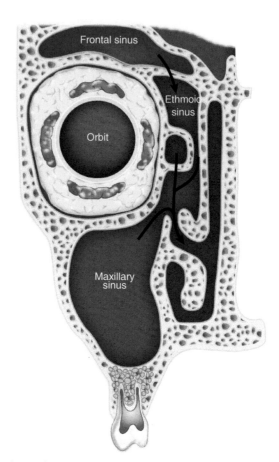

Fig. 3. Ostiomeatal complex.

Discharge; and Smell disorder. Minor symptoms that also help to support a diagnosis are cough, dental pain, ear pain/pressure, fatigue, halitosis, and headache. Generally, the presence of 2 major (PODS) criteria, or 1 major criterion and 2 minor criteria are diagnostic of acute sinusitis.[8] Other clinical criteria include the Williams and Berg criteria (**Table 3**).

Laboratory Tests

Erythrocyte sedimentation rate (ESR) and C-reactive protein (CRP) have been studied as diagnostic aids for ABRS, but in clinical practice, their role is not clearly defined. In

Table 1	
Sinusitis classification based on symptom duration	
Classification	**Symptom Duration**
Acute rhinosinusitis	<4 wk
Subacute rhinosinusitis	4–12 wk
Chronic rhinosinusitis	>12 wk
Recurrent rhinosinusitis	4 episodes/Yr without persistent symptoms in-between

Table 2
Special circumstances in sinusitis

Situation	History	Diagnosis/Pathogen	Treatment
Pilot or SCUBA diver	• Pain associated with pressure change • +/− epistaxis	• Sinus squeeze • Barosinusitis	• Decongestants • Intranasal steroids • Avoid pressure changes
Cystic fibrosis	• Acute or chronic sinusitis	• Pseudomonas • MRSA • Fungi	• Broad-spectrum coverage • ENT consultation
Older, diabetic patient	• Acute febrile illness • Dark nasal discharge • +/− DKA	• Mucormycosis, possible invasive infection	• Advanced imaging • IV antifungals • Surgical consultation
Recent dental procedure or infection	• Unilateral facial swelling and pain	• Odontogenic maxillary sinusitis • Polymicrobial	• OMFS ± ENT consultation • Broad-spectrum antibiotics • Anaerobic coverage
History of nasal vestibulitis with new symptoms of sinusitis	• Nare crusting, pain, and itching	• MRSA sinusitis	• MRSA coverage • Consider decolonizing treatment
Transplant Chemotherapy Severe immunocompromise	• Headache, facial pain, +/− fever, necrotic drainage	• Bacterial sinusitis • Fungal sinusitis	• Imaging • ENT consultation • IV antibiotics • Admit
Child with forehead pain and soft tissue swelling	• Fever, headache, upper respiratory symptoms	• Pott puffy tumor • Possible *Fusobacterium*	• Imaging • ENT consultation
ICU patient Recent intubation	• Fever, discharge, nasal drainage	• Polymicrobial infection • Possible *Pseudomonas*	• IV antibiotics • ENT consultation
Vertex headache	• Headache without facial pain	• Sphenoid sinusitis	• Consider cavernous sinus thrombosis • Image as indicated
Primary ciliary dyskinesis	• Recurrent pneumonia, Kartagener syndrome	• *Pseudomonas*	• Antibiotics • ENT referral

Abbreviations: DKA, diabetic ketoacidosis; ENT, otolaryngology; ICU, intensive care unit; IV, intravenous; MRSA, methicillin-resistant *Staphylococcus aureus*; OMFS, oral maxillofacial surgery.

Table 3
Comparison of acute rhinosinusitis diagnostic criteria

Berg Criteria[8,9]	Williams Criteria[10]	PODS Criteria[11]
Symptoms >7–10 d	Symptoms >7–10 d	Symptoms >7 d, worsening after 5–7 d, nasal purulence for 3–4 d with high fever
2 or more of the following	(+) 4 or more of the following (Intermediate) 2–3 (−) <2	≥2 of the following: Must have 1 of "O" or "D"
• Purulent rhinorrhea with unilateral predominance • Local pain with unilateral predominance • Bilateral purulent rhinorrhea • Pus in the nasal cavity	• Maxillary toothache • Purulent nasal secretion • History of colored nasal discharge • Poor response to nasal decongestants • Abnormal sinus transillumination	P Facial *Pain/Pressure* O Nasal *Obstruction* D *Discolored/purulent Discharge* S *Smell: Hyposmia or anosmia*
LR (3 or 4): 6.75 LR (0 or 1): 0.06	LR (+) = 4.7 LR (−) = 0.4	
Reference standard: sinus aspirate	Reference standard: sinus radiographs	Expert consensus only

Abbreviation: LR, likelihood ratio.

one study of 173 patients, 79% of those with a CRP greater than 49 mg/L had acute maxillary sinusitis compared with 61% with a CRP of 11 to 49 mg/L, and 34% of those with a CRP less than 11 mg/L.[12] An ESR less than 10 has been shown to have a negative likelihood ratio of 0.57, whereas an ESR greater than 40 has a positive likelihood ratio of 7.40. A single study suggested that testing nasal secretions for the presence of leukocyte esterase and nitrites with a urine dipstick was highly specific, and the absence of protein was highly sensitive, for ABRS.[12] Blood cultures are of minimal clinical utility in sinusitis and have poor correlation with cultures from sinus mucus.[13]

Imaging

Plain radiographs
Plain radiographs have been shown to correlate poorly with more sensitive sinus imaging techniques, such as computed tomography (CT) or MRI, and are no longer recommended in the evaluation of acute uncomplicated rhinosinusitis.[12,14]

Computed tomography/MRI
For patients with recurrent acute or chronic rhinosinusitis, or in whom symptoms persist after completing maximal medical therapy, CT of the sinuses without intravenous contrast is the imaging modality of choice. Opacification with fluid and thickened mucosa greater than 5 mm are suggestive of infection, but CT is not able to differentiate bacterial from viral or noninfectious etiologies. Studies also show findings consistent with sinusitis in up to 44% of adults and 50% of children imaged for unrelated reasons.[14] Sinus mucosal thickening can persist for 8 weeks following sinusitis despite treatment and symptom resolution.[15]

CT of the sinuses should be performed when there is a suspicion for orbital and intracranial complications of sinusitis.[3] However, MRI is superior for evaluating soft tissue and fluid densities, and the addition of gadolinium contrast can aid in identifying hyperemia, tumors, vascular anomalies, and intracranial extension of infection.[16]

Ultrasound

Ultrasonography can be used to evaluate for fluid in the sinuses and mucosal thickening. The clinical utility of routine ultrasound for the diagnosis of ABRS is poorly defined. A fluid-filled maxillary sinus, a "sinusogram," may suggest sinusitis, and may have greater utility in specific clinical situations, such as in patients in the intensive care unit.[17,18]

MICROBIOLOGY

Stagnant mucosal secretions act as a favorable medium for bacterial growth, yet only approximately one-third of sinus fluid aspirates in patients with suspected acute maxillary sinusitis are positive for bacterial pathogens.[12] ABRS has been classically caused by a triad of pathogens: *Streptococcus pneumoniae, Haemophilus influenzae B,* and *Moraxella catarrhalis*. However, there is great variability in the pathogenic causes of sinusitis, with anaerobes, gram-negative organisms, methicillin-resistant *Staphylococcus aureus* (MRSA), *Fusobacterium,* and polymicrobial and fungal pathogens all playing a role.[4] Distinguishing pathogens from colonizing bacteria can be difficult, especially in chronic rhinosinusitis. *Staphylococcus aureus* is present in the nasal flora of 20% to 30% of the healthy adult population, and MRSA in 3% to 6%. Fungi are almost universally present on cultures from patients with and without clinical signs of sinusitis.[19] Complicated rhinosinusitis is more closely associated with anaerobes (38.5%), *Streptococcus viridans* (34.6%), and staphylococcal species (30.8%).[20] The *Streptococcus milleri* group is commonly associated with abscess formation.[13]

There is evidence of a shift in pathogen prevalence since the widespread introduction of the pneumococcal conjugate vaccines.[13,21] Cultures from orbital complications of sinusitis decreased from 22% for *Streptococcus pneumoniae* and 12% for *S. viridans* in the prepneumococcal vaccine era to nearly zero in the postvaccine era. During this time, the number of cultures positive for *S. aureus* doubled, and half of these were MRSA. Hospitalization for sinusitis in children also decreased significantly in the postvaccine era.[13,22]

A recent large retrospective study evaluating the prevalence of MRSA in complicated pediatric rhinosinusitis found MRSA in 8% of surgical cultures; 75% of these infections grew MRSA alone, and 25% were polymicrobial. MRSA was associated with higher rates of intraorbital extension but low rates of intracranial infection.[23]

In chronic rhinosinusitis, anaerobic species, such as *Peptostreptococcus, Fusobacterium, Prevotella,* and *Propionibacterium*, are common.[24] With chronic sinusitis, the presence of nasal polyps is associated with higher rates of infection with *Staphylococcus, Alloiococcus, Corynebacterium* spp, and gram-negative infections.[6,25] The microbiology of odontogenic maxillary sinusitis differs from that of ABRS and commonly involves a mixed aerobic/anaerobic infection with pathogens including *Streptococcus, Bacteroides,* and *Proteus* spp, as well as coliform bacilli.[13,26] Noninvasive fungal disease includes fungus balls and allergic fungal rhinosinusitis, the latter of which is most often due to *Aspergillus flavus*.[27]

TREATMENT

Studies of ABRS treatment face many methodological challenges. The gold standard for diagnosis of ABRS is sinus meatus puncture with aspiration and culture, which is rarely done. A large percentage of patients with ABRS improve without any treatment, and many antibiotic prescriptions are unlikely to provide benefit. Expert recommendation, including the "Choosing Wisely" campaigns of emergency medicine, family medicine, and allergy and immunology, suggests that clinicians apply three principles in determining appropriate antibiotic prescriptions: assessing the likelihood of a bacterial infection, weighing benefits and harms of antibiotics, and implementing judicious prescribing strategies with regard to antibiotic selection and duration.[28,29]

Antibiotics

Evidence for benefit

Many randomized controlled trials have been performed to evaluate the efficacy of antibiotics in the treatment of ABRS. An important finding is the high rate of symptom improvement in patients receiving placebo, consistently occurring in 60% to 80%. This contributes to a relatively low measured benefit of antibiotics.[4,30,31] Failure to identify patients who meet strict diagnostic criteria for sinusitis will lead to an even lower measured benefit. A pediatric study using strict diagnostic criteria found improvement in 32% of patients who received placebo and 64% of those who received antibiotics.[32]

Meta-analyses of randomized controlled trials show only a 7% to 14% higher rate of cure or improvement between 7 and 15 days with antibiotics compared with placebo.[33] A greater benefit is observed for preventing worsening of symptoms than for symptom resolution. Some, but not all, studies have shown that antibiotics shorten symptom duration by 2 to 3 days.[34,35] The rate of complications and recurrence do not differ. Adverse effects, primarily diarrhea, are 80% more common with antibiotics.[4,29] The overall number needed to harm has been estimated at 8, although most side effects are minor and self-limited.[36] There is no demonstrated benefit of antibiotics for preventing suppurative complications of sinusitis.[4] Treatment of chronic rhinosinusitis requires a prolonged courses of antibiotics of up to 3 months to achieve minor and transient benefits.[19]

In general, antibiotics should be reserved for patients with clear clinical signs of ABRS who present with severe symptoms, such as high fever, do not show improvement after 10 days of conservative therapy, or acutely worsen after an initial period of improvement. Antibiotics also should be considered in patients with immunocompromise, mucociliary dysfunction, or other risk factors for poor outcome.

Antibiotic selection

Amoxicillin with or without clavulanic acid is the preferred first-line therapy for sinusitis. The addition of a β-lactamase inhibitor has been associated with slightly higher rates of cure. Due to increased resistance of S. pneumoniae and H influenzae to azithromycin, second-generation and third-generation cephalosporins, and trimethoprim-sulfamethoxazole, these agents are no longer recommended as first-line agents.

Treatment failure (worsening symptoms or failure of response at 7 days) should prompt clinicians to consider second-line therapeutic options (**Table 4**).[31,37] Respiratory fluoroquinolones should be reserved for patients without other therapeutic options or those with suspected pseudomonal infection (eg, patients with cystic fibrosis), due to higher rates of adverse effects. Patients treated with first-line and second-line antibiotics both have cure rates of more than 90%.[38,39]

Duration

The recommended duration of antibiotic therapy for ABRS is between 5 and 10 days. A meta-analysis looking at duration of antibiotic therapy within the recommended range found no difference in outcome between short courses of 5 days and longer courses. Patients with complicating factors, such as immunosuppression or chronic underlying diseases, are excluded from most studies and should not be considered candidates for shorter courses of therapy.[40]

Table 4			
Acute bacterial rhinosinusitis antibiotic regimens			
Treatment	**General**	**Penicillin Allergy**	**Pediatric**
First line	Amoxicillin ± clavulanic acid	Doxycycline Clindamycin + (cefixime or cefpodoxime)	Amoxicillin ± clavulanic acid
Second line	Amoxicillin + clavulanic acid (high dose) Doxycycline Clindamycin + (cefixime or cefpodoxime) Levofloxacin or moxifloxacin	Clindamycin + (cefixime or cefpodoxime) (if doxycycline failure) Levofloxacin or moxifloxacin	Amoxicillin + clavulanic acid (high dose) Clindamycin + (cefixime or cefpodoxime) Doxycycline (age >8 y)

Intranasal Steroids and Other Therapies

Intranasal steroids, including budesonide, mometasone, and fluticasone, may be effective as monotherapy in the treatment of acute rhinosinusitis to reduce inflammation, mucus secretion, facial pain, and congestion.[41,42] Benefit may require up to 3 weeks to be detected and there is a dose-response relationship with the greatest benefit seen with higher doses.[43] Intranasal corticosteroids appear to have greater benefit in patients with a history of allergic rhinitis.[37] There is no evidence of significant adverse events related to intranasal steroids.

Sinonasal saline irrigation assists in removing mucus and environmental irritants and restoring normal mucociliary function. A 2007 Cochrane review showed that daily nasal irrigation with isotonic or hypertonic saline decreased symptoms of sinusitis, but a subsequent review in 2010 challenged this conclusion. The potential benefit of saline irrigation appears to be greater when used in combination with intranasal steroids and/or antibiotics than when used as single therapy.[3,37,43]

There is no convincing evidence that decongestants or antihistamines are effective in the treatment of acute rhinosinusitis.[37] If decongestants are used, topical administration is preferred to systemic, and duration of therapy should be limited to 72 hours.[44] Over-the-counter analgesics, such as acetaminophen or nonsteroidal anti-inflammatory drugs, are safe and effective for pain associated with sinusitis. Opioid analgesics are not recommended due to potential for adverse events.

Treatment Summary

Initial treatment for undifferentiated rhinosinusitis can include intranasal steroids, saline irrigation, and analgesics. Antibiotics should be reserved for patients with symptoms that are persistent and not improving at 10 days, worsening symptoms at any time after diagnosis, or severe symptoms. Severe symptoms include fever ≥39°C and/or purulent nasal discharge for at least 3 days.[28] Empiric antibiotic coverage should be first-line antibiotics such as amoxicillin. It is not necessary to cover routinely for MRSA.[37]

COMPLICATIONS

Complications of ABRS are rare but can be severe. Complications are divided anatomically into intracranial complications and extracranial complications. The estimated rate of complications of ABRS is only 1 in 1000 cases.[12]

Intracranial Complications

Sinusitis is the single leading cause of intracranial abscess. Epidural abscess is the most common intracranial complication of sinusitis followed by subdural empyema.[45] Intracranial seeding of infection is believed to occur primarily via septic emboli transmitted through valveless diploic veins in the skull base, which penetrate the dura. Seeding can also occur via direct extension of osteomyelitis, or through bony defects or skull ostia.

Intracranial complications are more likely to arise from frontal or ethmoid sinusitis.[45,46] One study found that 60% of patients with a sinogenic epidural abscess also had osteomyelitis of the posterior table of the frontal bone.[6] Sphenoid sinusitis occurs in only 3% of cases of ABRS, and usually in the setting of pansinusitis, but is associated with parietal and temporal lobe abscesses and meningitis.[47] Maxillary sinusitis has the lowest association with suppurative complications.[45]

Intracranial complications are more common in children than in adults, with a peak age near 13 years.[23] These conditions have been observed in 3% to 4% of sinusitis cases serious enough to be admitted to the hospital.

Only a small percentage of patients with intracranial complications will have previously been diagnosed with sinusitis. Fewer than half of patients present with any neurologic deficit, and the presence of neurologic deficit is most common with subdural empyema, meningitis, or CST. Epidural abscess, the most common intracranial complication, frequently presents without neurologic deficits, and more commonly presents with pain referred to the eye and forehead.[6]

MRI has been found to be superior to CT in diagnosing intracranial complications of sinusitis, with reported sensitivities of 93% versus 63%.[6] Few clinical findings correlate well with intracranial complications, but neurologic deficits and orbital symptoms warrant liberal imaging. More than half of cultures from patients with intracranial complications grow multiple organisms. *Streptococcus milleri* is the single most common bacterial isolate in children with intracranial abscesses. Gram-negative rods account for approximately 10% of isolates.[46]

CST is associated with a number of craniofacial infections, including sphenoid and ethmoid sinusitis. It frequently presents with spiking fevers, orbital pain, and headache, and progresses to cause proptosis, ophthalmoplegia, visual impairment, and cranial nerve palsies. Cranial nerve VI is most commonly involved, due to its location within the cavernous sinus. Cranial nerves III, IV, V1, and V2 can be affected due to their proximity to the lateral wall of the sinus[45] (see **Fig. 2**).

Treatment of all intracranial complications involves intravenous antibiotics and surgical consultation for possible drainage. Intravenous antibiotics should be broad-spectrum, covering MRSA, oral anaerobes, and the classic triad of acute sinusitis organisms (*Streptococcus pneumoniae, Haemophilus influenzae B*, and *Moraxella catarrhalis*).[23] There is controversy regarding the use of corticosteroids in the setting of intracranial abscess, as no evidence exists to show benefit, even when cerebral edema is present.[45]

Despite aggressive treatment of intracranial complications, mortality rates are 10% to 20%.[46] Among survivors, significant long-term disability is frequent, with 13% to 35% of patients experiencing hemiparesis, aphasia, hydrocephalus, epilepsy, and/or visual defects.[45]

Extracranial Complications

Extracranial complications of sinusitis include orbital cellulitis or abscess, Pott puffy tumor, and mucoceles. Orbital complications of sinusitis are more common than intracranial complications and occur more commonly in children, with a peak incidence in the first decade of life.[23]

Orbital infections are most frequently associated with infection of the posterior ethmoid sinuses or the maxillary sinuses.[13] Infection can spread from the ethmoid sinus to the orbit directly through the lamina papyracea. Infection can also spread inferiorly into the orbit from the frontal sinus.[45] A significant proportion of adults with orbital complications of sinusitis have diabetes mellitus, and these patients are more likely to have advanced stages of infection.[48]

Pott's puffy tumor is a subperiosteal abscess due to osteomyelitis of the anterior table of the frontal sinus. In addition to headache and fever, fluctuant swelling of the forehead is characteristic. Treatment includes intravenous antibiotics and surgical drainage with debridement of necrotic bone. Despite being extracranial, there is a 60% to 85% association of Pott's puffy tumor with simultaneous intracranial complications.

Mucoceles of the paranasal sinuses are chronic, benign, and expansile lesions filled with mucus and epithelial cells. They develop most commonly in the frontal sinus as a result of obstruction from inflammation or trauma. A mucocele can become secondarily infected and form an abscess, known as a mucopyocele. Mucoceles also can cause bony erosion of the walls of the sinus and have the potential to extend intracranially or into the orbit, causing infection or mass effect.[45]

INVASIVE CRANIOFACIAL FUNGAL RHINOSINUSITIS

Fungal rhinosinusitis can lead to acute or chronic invasive disease. Chronic fungal sinusitis can occur in immunocompetent hosts. Acute invasive fungal sinusitis occurs almost exclusively in immunocompromised hosts, is rapidly progressive, and has high mortality. It is most frequently caused by *Aspergillus* in patients with hematological malignancies, whereas *Mucor* and *Rhizopus* more often cause disease in diabetic patients. Acute fungal infection is invasive and can spread into any adjacent anatomic structure. Intracranial spread can lead to seizures, altered mental status, cranial neuropathies, or focal neurologic deficits. Treatment requires aggressive surgical debridement and intravenous antifungal therapy. If fungal invasion reaches the central nervous system, mortality rates are 40% to 80%.[45]

SUMMARY

Sinusitis is a challenging clinical problem with substantial ongoing debate regarding diagnosis and treatment. Emergency providers need to be familiar with several special circumstances to tailor treatment and achieve optimal outcomes. Extensive literature on sinusitis emphasizes the following key points:

- Rhinosinusitis can be allergic, viral, bacterial, fungal, or barotraumatic in etiology.
- Laboratory studies, cultures of the nasopharynx or blood, and radiologic imaging are not indicated in the workup of uncomplicated ABRS.
- Pneumococcal conjugate vaccine has reduced the rate of streptococcal sinus infection, but streptococci remain important pathogens.
- Most cases of ABRS will resolve without antibiotics.
- Strict clinical diagnostic criteria should be used to identify cases of ABRS requiring antibiotics.
- Amoxicillin, with or without clavulanic acid, is the first-line therapeutic choice for ABRS; duration of treatment is 5 to 10 days.
- Intranasal steroids are useful alone or with antibiotics, especially when allergic inflammation is believed to be a causative factor.

- Nasal irrigation with saline solution may provide symptomatic relief.
- Patients with diabetes mellitus, asthma, cystic fibrosis, severe dental disease, immunocompromise, and ciliary dyskinesis are predisposed to complicated rhinosinusitis.
- Intracranial and extracranial complications of sinusitis are associated with substantial morbidity and mortality, and are diagnosed with MRI or CT.
- If rhinosinusitis is recurrent or chronic, referral for allergy testing and evaluation for nasal polyps is recommended.

REFERENCES

1. Ray NF, Baraniuk JN, Thamer M, et al. Healthcare expenditures for sinusitis in 1996: contributions of asthma, rhinitis, and other airway disorders. J Allergy Clin Immunol 1999;103:408–14.
2. Lethbridge-Cejku M, Schiller JS, Bernadel L. Summary health statistics for U.S. adults: National Health Interview Survey, 2002. Vital Health Stat 10 2004;(222): 1–151.
3. Wald E, Applegate K, Bordley C, et al. Clinical practice guidelines for the diagnosis and management of acute bacterial sinusitis in children aged 1 to 18 years. Pediatrics 2013;132(1):e262–80.
4. Falagas M, Giannapoulou K, Vardakas KZ, et al. Comparison of antibiotics with placebo for treatment of acute sinusitis: a meta-analysis of randomized control trials. Lancet Infect Dis 2008;8:543–52.
5. Battisti AS, Lark JD. Barosinusitis. [Updated 2018 Sep 9]. In: StatPearls [Internet]. Treasure Island (FL): StatPearls Publishing; 2018. Available at: https://www.ncbi.nlm.nih.gov/books/NBK470207/.
6. Niederfuhr A, Kirsche H, Riechelmann H, et al. The bacteriology of rhinosinusitis with and without nasal polyps. Arch Otolaryngol Head Neck Surg 2009;135(2): 131–6.
7. Rosenfeld RM, Piccirillo JF, Chandrasekhar SS, et al. Clinical practice guidelines (update): adult sinusitis. Otolaryngol Head Neck Surg 2015;152(2 suppl):S1–39.
8. Kaplan A. Canadian guidelines for acute bacterial rhinosinusitis. Can Fam Physician 2014;60:227–34.
9. Berg O, Carenfelt C. Analysis of symptoms and clinical signs in the maxillary sinus empyema. Acta Otolaryngol 1988;105(3–4):343–9.
10. Williams JW, Simel DL, Roberts L, et al. Clinical evaluation of sinusitis: making the diagnosis by history and physical examination. Ann Intern Med 1992;117(9): 705–10.
11. Desrosiers M, Evans GA, Keith PK, et al. Canadian clinical practice guidelines for acute and chronic rhinosinusitis. J Otolaryngol Head Neck Surg 2011;40(S2): S99–193.
12. Aring A, Chan M. Acute rhinosinusitis in adults. Am Fam Physician 2016;94(2): 97–105.
13. Peña M, Preciado D, Orestes M, et al. Orbital complications of acute sinusitis: changes in the post-pneumococcal vaccine era. JAMA Otolaryngol Head Neck Surg 2013;139(3):223–7.
14. Manning S, Biavati M, Phillips DL. Correlation of clinical sinusitis signs and symptoms to imaging findings in pediatric patients. Int J Pediatr Otorhinolaryngol 1996;37:65–74.
15. Leopold DA, Stafford CT, Sod EW, et al. Clinical course of acute maxillary sinusitis documented by sequential MRI scanning. Am J Rhinol 1994;8:19928.

16. Fatterpekar GM, Delman BN, Som PM. Imaging the paranasal sinuses: where are we and where are we going? Anat Rec 2008;291:1564–72.
17. Ebell M, McKay B, Guibault R, et al. Diagnosis of acute rhinosinusitis in primary care: a systematic review of test accuracy. Br J Gen Pract 2016;66(650):e612–32.
18. Lichtenstein D, Biderman P, Mezière G, et al. The "sinusogram", a real-time ultrasound sign of maxillary sinusitis. Intensive Care Med 1998;24:1057–61.
19. Barshak MB, Durand ML. The role of infection and antibiotics in chronic rhinosinusitis. Laryngoscope Investig Otolaryngol 2017;2(1):36–42.
20. Brook I. Bacteriology of chronic sinusitis and acute exacerbation of chronic sinusitis. Arch Otolaryngol Head Neck Surg 2006;132:1099–101.
21. Kosteniemi U, Palm J, Silfverdal S. Reductions in otitis and other respiratory tract infections following childhood pneumococcal vaccination. Acta Paediatr 2018. https://doi.org/10.1111/apa.14345.
22. Lindstrand A, Bennel R, Galanis I, et al. Sinusitis and pneumonia hospitalization after introduction of pneumococcal conjugate vaccine. Pediatrics 2014;134(6): e1528–36.
23. Hamill C, Sykes K, Harrison C, et al. Infection rates of MRSA in complicated pediatric rhinosinusitis: an up to date review. Int J Pediatr Otorhinolaryngol 2018; 104:79–83.
24. Ramadan H. What is the bacteriology of chronic sinusitis in adults? Am J Otolaryngol 1995;16(5):303–6.
25. Lal D, Keim P, Delisle J, et al. Mapping and comparing bacterial microbiota in the sinonasal cavity of healthy, allergic rhinitis, and chronic rhinosinusitis subjects. Int Forum Allergy Rhinol 2017;7(6):561–9.
26. Saibene A, Vassena C, Pipolo C, et al. Odontogenic and rhinogenic chronic sinusitis: a modern microbiological comparison. Int Forum Allergy Rhinol 2016; 6(1):41–5.
27. Singh A, Gupta P, Verma N, et al. Fungal rhinosinusitis: microbiological and histopathological perspective. J Clin Diagn Res 2017;11(7):DC10–2.
28. Hersh A, Jackson M, Hicks L, et al. Principles of judicious antibiotic prescribing for upper respiratory tract infections in pediatrics. Pediatrics 2013;132(6): 1146–54.
29. Smith S, Montgomery L, Williams J. Treatment of mild to moderate sinusitis. Arch Intern Med 2012;172(6):510–3.
30. Buchem F, Knottnerus J, Schrijnemaekers V, et al. Primary-care-based placebo-controlled trial of antibiotic treatment in acute maxillary sinusitis. Lancet 1997; 349:683–7.
31. Stalman W, Van Essen G, Van der Graaf Y, et al. The end of antibiotic treatment in adults with acute sinusitis-like complaints in general practice? A placebo-controlled, double-blind randomized doxycycline trial. Br J Gen Pract 1997;47: 794–9.
32. Wald E, Nash D, Eickhoff J. Effectiveness of amoxicillin/clavulanate potassium in the treatment of acute bacterial sinusitis in children. Pediatrics 2009;124(1):9–15.
33. Ahovuo-Salvoranta A, Borisenko OV, Kovanen N, et al. Antibiotics for acute maxillary sinusitis. Cochrane Database Syst Rev 2008;(2):CD000243.
34. Merenstein D, Whittaker C, Chadwell T, et al. Are antibiotics beneficial for sinusitis complaints? J Fam Pract 2005;54(2):144–51.
35. Williamson I, Rumsby K, Benge S, et al. Antibiotics and topical nasal steroids for treatment of acute maxillary sinusitis: a randomized control trial. JAMA 2007; 298(21):2487–96.

36. Lemiengre MB, van Driel ML, Merenstrin D, et al. Antibiotics for clinically diagnosed acute rhinosinusitis in adults. Cochrane Database Syst Rev 2012;(10):CD006089.
37. Chow A, Benninger M, Brook I, et al. IDSA clinical practice guideline for acute bacterial rhinosinusitis in children and adults. Clin Infect Dis 2012;54:1041–5.
38. Piccirillo J, Mager D, Frisse M, et al. Impact of first-line vs. second-line antibiotics for the treatment of acute uncomplicated sinusitis. JAMA 2001;286(15):1849–56.
39. Karageorgopolous D, Giannopoulou K, Grammatikos AP, et al. Fluoroquinolones compared with B-lactam antibiotics for the treatment of acute bacterial sinusitis: a meta-analysis of randomized control trials. CMAJ 2008;178(7):845–54.
40. Falagas M, Karageorgopolous D, Grammatikos A, et al. Effectiveness and safety of short vs. long duration of antibiotic therapy for acute bacterial sinusitis: a meta-analysis of randomized control trials. Br J Clin Pharmacol 2009;67(2):161–71.
41. Blin P, Blazejewski S, Severine L, et al. Effectiveness of antibiotics for acute sinusitis in real-life medical practice. Br J Clin Pharmacol 2010;70(3):418–28.
42. Hayward G, Heneghan C, Perera R, et al. Intranasal corticosteroids in management of acute sinusitis: review and metaanalysis. Ann Fam Med 2012;10(3):241–9.
43. Rudmik L, Soler Z. Medical therapies for adult chronic sinusitis: a systematic review. JAMA 2015;314(9):926–39.
44. McCormick D, John S, Swischuk L, et al. A double-blind, placebo-controlled trial of decongestant-antihistamine for the treatment of sinusitis in children. Clin Pediatr 1996;35(9):457–60.
45. Ziegler A, Patadia M, Stankiewicz J. Neurological complications of acute and chronic sinusitis. Curr Neurol Neurosci Rep 2018;18(2):5.
46. Germiller J, Monin D, Sparano AL, et al. Intracranial complications of sinusitis in children and adolescents and their outcomes. Arch Otolaryngol Head Neck Surg 2006;132:969–76.
47. Saitoh A, Beall B, Nizet V. Fulminant bacterial meningitis complicating sphenoid sinusitis. Pediatr Emerg Care 2003;19(6):415–7.
48. Chang YS, Chen PL, Hung JH, et al. Orbital complications of paranasal sinusitis in Taiwan, 1988 through 2015: acute ophthalmological manifestations, diagnosis, and management. PLoS One 2017;12(10):e0184477.

Soft Tissue Disorders of the Mouth

Stephanie Diebold, MD[a], Michael Overbeck, MD[b],*

KEYWORDS

- Candidiasis • Dental caries • Herpes labialis • Sialolithiasis • Oral lichen planus
- Aphthous ulcer • Oral leukoplakia • Mucocele

KEY POINTS

- Oral candidiasis is effectively treated with antifungal medications and may raise suspicion for an immunocompromised patient.
- If unrecognized or untreated, dental infections may extend into the floor of the mouth, the pharyngeal space, or mediastinum.
- When recognized, the duration and intensity of symptoms of herpes labialis can be decreased with antiviral medications.
- Premalignant or potentially malignant conditions, such as oral lichen planus or oral leukoplakia, should be recognized and referred by the emergency provider to prevent the rare but serious complications of malignant transformation.
- Common and generally benign lesions of the mouth are encountered by the emergency physician and include mucoceles and bony tori.

INTRODUCTION

Emergency providers encounter a wide range of pathologic and nonpathologic conditions of the mouth. Even in patients who have no stated concerns about the health of the mouth, clinicians routinely discover several common abnormalities, with varying impact on the ultimate diagnosis and management. This work discusses commonly observed conditions affecting the soft tissues of the mouth, generally reviewed in 3 categories:

1. Infectious processes, including oral candidiasis, herpes labialis, and general comments about the pathophysiology of dental caries and their complications

Disclosure Statement: Authors state no disclosures.
[a] Department of Emergency Medicine, Denver Health Hospital, 777 Bannock Street, MC #0108, Denver, CO 80204, USA; [b] Department of Emergency Medicine, University of Colorado School of Medicine, Denver, CO, USA
* Corresponding author. Leprino Office Building 712 Mail Stop B-215, 12401 East 17th Avenue, Aurora, CO 80045.
E-mail address: michael.overbeck@ucdenver.edu

Emerg Med Clin N Am 37 (2019) 55–68
https://doi.org/10.1016/j.emc.2018.09.006
0733-8627/19/© 2018 Elsevier Inc. All rights reserved.
emed.theclinics.com

2. Painful noninfectious conditions, including sialolithiasis, oral lichen planus (OLP), aphthous ulcer (AU), and oral leukoplakia
3. Benign conditions that, although clearly abnormal, pose little concern to the clinician or patient. This area includes mucoceles and bony tori.

INFECTIOUS PROCESSES
Oral Candidiasis

Etiology
Commonly referred to as thrush, oral candidiasis is found in young infants, older adults with dentures, patients using antibiotics, asthmatics that use inhaled glucocorticoids, and those in an immunodeficient state (chemotherapy, radiation, HIV/AIDS, or diabetes).[1] The etiologic agent is the yeast Candida albicans.

Clinical presentation
Thrush is most commonly seen as a pseudomembranous appearance with white plaques on the tongue, lips, palate, or buccal mucosa (**Fig. 1**) but can also appear as a atrophic form without plaques and only an erythematous appearance, commonly found beneath dentures.[1] Additionally, thrush can be seen as a bright red, painful tongue. Most oropharyngeal lesions are asymptomatic, although some patients may complain of dry mouth or pain.

Diagnosis
Diagnosis can be confirmed by scraping the lesion with a tongue depressor and performing a potassium hydroxide preparation where budding yeast are visible with or without pseudohyphae. If the lesions can be easily scraped off with a tongue depressor, if there is no systemic involvement, and if the presentation is both

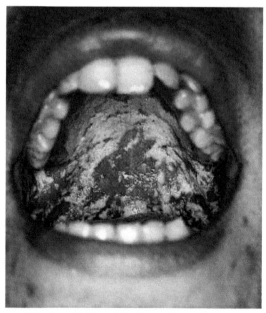

Fig. 1. White plaques of oral candidiasis (which can be scraped off to reveal an erythematous base) in an HIV-positive patient. (*Reprinted from* Hutchison's Clinical Methods: An Integrated Approach to Clinical Practice, 24th ed, John Peters, James Green, Lina Hijazi Urogenital system, pages 355–377, ©2018, with permission from Elsevier.)

historically and clinically consistent with typical *Candida*, however, basic treatment can be initiated and no formal method of diagnosis is necessary.

Treatment
If symptomatic, topical or systemic treatment may be needed.[2] Topical antifungal therapy is considered the treatment of basic candidiasis. Nystatin is the treatment of choice but clotrimazole also can be used. More specifically, nystatin 400,000 units to 600,000 units 4 times a day swish and swallow is used or a 10-mg lozenge of clotrimazole dissolved between the cheek and the gum 5 times daily. Candidiasis that is recurrent should bring up concern for possible immunodeficiency (HIV). Finally, fastidious and regular denture care should provide a basis for prevention.[3]

Dental Caries

Background
Dental caries is the most common cause of pain in the mouth.[3] Western countries have increased rates of caries compared with developed countries secondary to increased intake of refined sugars. Dental caries affects 91% of adults in the United States and is 5 times as common as asthma in children, making it the most prevalent pediatric disease.[4]

Etiology
Dental caries encompasses a continuous disease process mediated by dietary and host factors resulting in loss of dentin. The balance of host protective factors with the disease-causing biofilm development determines the extent and progression of the disease.[5] This balance is further influenced by fluctuations in degrees of demineralization and remineralization that occur throughout life.[6] The complex oral environment is dynamic and favors a constantly changing array of chemical and microbiological factors. If oral hygiene or dietary intake varies for even a few weeks (extended trips or hospitalization as examples), the process of dental caries can accelerate.[7] When pH of the oral environment drops below 5, demineralization is favored. As demineralization occurs, material is irretrievably lost and cavities form in the enamel. Groups of bacteria that influence and facilitate a low pH environment are the classic *Streptococcus mutans* and *Lactobacilli,* as well as acidogenic species, such as nonmutans *Streptococcus* and *Actinomyces.* Host factors that influence the physical environment, thereby increasing populations of cariogenic organisms, include frequent carbohydrate delivery (sugar consumption) and dehydration (leading to poor salivary flow and decreased pH buffering by reduced presence of saliva). Proliferation of these species forms a supragingival biofilm (dominated by gram-positive organisms) that perpetuates a microenvironment of low pH with demineralization. Host factors that influence caries formation are summarized in **Table 1**. The subgingival microbiome is dominated by gram-negative bacteria (*Actinobacillus, Fusobacterium*, and *Campylobacter* species, as examples) and causes periodontal disease and gingivitis. These constituents of oral flora have implications for the emergency physician in treating oral infections and extraoral infections believed attributable to poor oral hygiene (aspiration pneumonia or endocarditis).

Treatment
The mainstay treatment of dental caries is restorative intervention; however, more important are the primary preventive measures (see **Table 1**).

Complications
An apical abscess (also referred to as odontogenic abscess, dentoalveolar abscess, or simply dental abscess) is formed by a collection of bacteria, inflammatory

Table 1
Factors contributing to development of dental caries

Personal	Behavior Education oral health literacy Sociodemographic status, income Dental insurance coverage Knowledge attitudes	Twice-daily brushing significantly reduces risk Limit snacking Parental modeling and education Programs targeting low-income and underuninsured populations, with education of at-risk demographic groups
Oral environment	Saliva Sugars Protein Calcium, phosphate Plaque pH, antibacterial agents Chewing gum, fluoride, dental sealants	Hydration, balanced diet Limit processed sugar intake Regular dental examinations, twice-daily brushing with approved paste; occasional treatment with chlorhexidine as directed by dental professional Sugar-free chewing gum, fluoride topically via foods, water, dental products
Direct contributing	Diet Tooth Time Bacterial biofilm	Fermentable carbohydrates are metabolized by bacterial flora to generate organic acids, which favor demineralization. Primary teeth with plaque on maxillary incisors age 1 risk for future caries; first and second molars most susceptible First few years after tooth eruption are highest risk Combination of above factors can limit establishment of biofilm that favors local acidic pH, demineralization, dentin structure breakdown, ultimately requiring surgical intervention/restoration or, in some cases, removal

Additional details, see Refs.[45–49]

From Mejare I, Axelsson S, Dahlen G, et al. Caries risk assessment. A systematic review. Acta Odontol Scand 2014;72(2):81–91.

components, and cellular debris in a contained space characterized by liquefactive necrosis. Abscesses typically form after bacteria reach the dental pulp through chronic infection, caries, or trauma. Acute inflammation of apical periodontitis occurs at a rate of 5% per year,[8] is characterized by pain and swelling, and provides evidence of advanced stages of infection.

The clinical presentation of apical abscess is typically pain, swelling, occasional trismus, and lymphadenopathy. The affected tooth is frequently tender to percussion. Fever and headache are variably present. The evolution of an odontogenic abscess into a subcutaneous abscess results from the erosion of medullary and cortical bone to provide an egress of inflammatory components and formation of a soft tissue abscess. This process can extend into adjacent areas, such as the floor of the mouth (sublingual space), the neck (submandibular, pterygomandibular, and parapharyngeal spaces), or face (maxillary sinus, masseteric, and buccal spaces). Bilateral involvement of the sublingual and submandibular spaces is characterized by tenderness and firmness across the midline, limited tongue movement and absence of lymphadenopathy, raising concern for the uncommon necrotizing infectious condition known as Ludwig angina (attributed to the description by Wilhelm Frederick von Ludwig in 1836 combined with the Latin, *angere*, meaning *to strangle*).[9] Although imaging may clarify the presence of gas or fluid collections in the floor of the mouth or neck, the diagnosis of Ludwig's angina is clinical. The location and feared natural course of this condition jeopardize the airway patency and can be fatal if not managed promptly with broad-spectrum antibiotics and surgical consultation. A considered approach in managing the airway is mandatory because several markers of the anatomically difficult airway are typically present (tongue swelling, trismus, pharyngeal edema, and inflammation). Experienced providers typically opt for fiberoptic or videolaryngoscopic techniques in managing the airway to insure successful endotracheal intubation on the first attempt. Although rare, further spread into deep spaces can result in cavernous sinus thrombosis, brain abscess, epidural abscess, and necrotizing infections—although these are infrequent enough to rise to the level of case reports.[7] Odontogenic abscess presenting to the emergency department can often be managed with primary incision and drainage. Given a normal host response to infection, most locally contained abscesses can be managed without antibiotics. Should antibiotics be deemed necessary, empiric penicillin V, amoxicillin (with or without clavulanate), or clindamycin in patients with an established penicillin allergy are typically first line. Anti-inflammatories are typically used on a scheduled basis for swelling and pain for the first 2 days to 3 days after incision and drainage or institution of antibiotics. Immediate-release opiate prescriptions are deemphasized given the risk to the patient, risk of diversion, and typical single-encounter nature of the physician-patient relationship characteristic of emergency medicine. Opiates remain an important tool in managing pain, however, and a strategy including opiates may be used on a case by case basis.[10]

Herpes Labialis

Etiology
Also called oral herpes or cold sores, herpes labialis is caused by the herpes simplex virus (HSV) type 1, affecting 2 in 3 adults worldwide.[11] Primary exposure to HSV-1 results from perioral exposure in early childhood and often manifests as a mild or even subclinical event. Recurrent oral HSV-1 infection is termed, *herpes labialis*.

Clinical presentation
Herpes labialis lesions are vesicular eruptions on or adjacent to the lip and recur variably, from minor nuisance occurring infrequently, to monthly or more frequent outbreaks with prominent painful lesions about the lips and oral mucosa. Herpes labialis has the appearance of a vesicular lesion with an erythematous base often presenting as multiple grouped lesions (**Fig. 2**). HSV-1 persists in the neural ganglia and recurs for various reasons, including sun exposure, stress, infection, or trauma.

Treatment
The decision to treat this painful condition is complicated by lack of demonstrably effective therapy. Several clinical trials have found that little benefit is conveyed unless therapy is initiated within the first 2 days.[12–16] If patients can detect the prodromal symptoms early, topical or oral treatment can have some therapeutic effect. This type of treatment approach is considered episodic treatment, where the patient is responsible to detect prodromal symptoms and treat the specific episode when it occurs.

Topical therapy with either acyclovir or penciclovir demonstrated minimal impact on symptoms (duration of pain and vesicle appearance decreased by less than

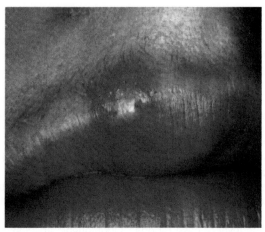

Fig. 2. Clinical presentation of herpes labialis on the mucocutaneous junction of the upper lip. (*From* Samaranayake L. Viruses of relevance to dentistry. In: Samaranayake L, ed. Essential Microbiology for Dentistry. 5th ed. Philadelphia, PA: Elsevier; 2018: 175–186; with permission.)

1 day).[12,15] Oral therapy shows similarly modest advantages in controlled trials. For example, acyclovir versus placebo was seen to decrease the duration of lesions by approximately 2.1 days if taken within 1 hour of prodromal symptom onset.[14] Furthermore, valacyclovir also shortens the duration of recurrent episodes by approximately 1 day versus placebo.[14] Both valacyclovir and famciclovir have increased oral bioavailability and they are taken with less frequency than acyclovir; however, they tend to be much more expensive than acyclovir.[15,17]

Another treatment approach consists of treating regularly to prevent recurrent episodes, or chronic suppressive treatment. This type of approach is considered for individuals with frequent recurrence or severe symptoms. Several trials have shown that when taken on a daily basis, both use of acyclovir and valacyclovir reduce the number of outbreaks.[18–21]

Currently, there is no preventive vaccine available for recurrent herpes labialis. Research studying the effects of herpes glycoproteins (specifically glycoprotein D) has demonstrated success in eliciting T-cell–mediated immunity in animal models.[22] Development of epitopes specific to HSV-1 and HSV-2 glycoprotein D may elicit immune response from both CD-4 and CD-8 T cells, potentially conveying immunity.[23] Attenuated viruses do elicit humoral and cellular responses and may provide a route to vaccine development.[24]

PAINFUL NONINFECTIOUS PROCESSES
Sialolithiasis

Etiology
Salivary stones are caused by stasis of saliva and inflammation of the salivary ducts and can be complicated by superimposed infection. Predisposing factors to salivary stone formation include medications, dehydration, and malnutrition.

Clinical presentation
The most common location for formation of salivary stones is in the submandibular duct, or Wharton duct (**Fig. 3**). It is believed that the upward course of saliva from the inferior position of the gland to the more superior exit to the floor of the mouth predisposes to

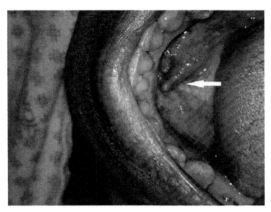

Fig. 3. Right submandibular swelling caused by sialolithiasis in Wharton duct (*arrow*) with resultant sialadenitis. (*From* Huang F, Caton R, Colla J. Point-of-care ultrasound diagnosis of acute sialolithiasis with sialadenitis. Clin Pract Cases Emerg Med 2017;1(4):437; with permission.)

stasis of the saliva.[25] The second most common location for sialoliths is the parotid duct, or Stensen duct. Calcium carbonate and calcium phosphate make up a majority of stones. Sialolithiasis usually presents as sudden pain, irritation, and inflammation in a salivary gland around the time of eating and are more common in women in the sixth decade of life.[26] The salivary stone is often visualized with direct view or by milking the gland on examination. There is only overlying erythema or visible pus when there is a superimposed infection of the stone. To confirm the diagnosis, if the stone is not visualized grossly on examination, imaging can be helpful. Plain radiographs obtained from an anteroposterior orientation with mouth open and chin extended can detect submandibular stones.[27] With recent emphasis on speed, cost, and radiation exposure, ultrasonography is becoming more widely available and utilized. Extraoral and now intraoral ultrasonography has been shown to detect stones greater than 2 mm in size with high sensitivity.[28,29] When the diagnosis remains in question, CT, obtained without contrast, has a high sensitivity in detecting sialolithiases.[27]

Treatment

If the stone is visible and can be milked out of the gland with sequential bimanual pressure along the occluded duct, this is an effective method for salivary stone expulsion in addition to hydration, anti-inflammatories, and sialagogues like sour candy or vitamin C lozenges. If stone removal is necessary and sequential external pressure is unsuccessful, a ductal papillary incision can be performed. This procedure is typically performed by an oral surgeon. Antibiotics are not necessary unless the duct obstruction has resulted in infectious inflammation of the salivary gland, termed *sialadenitis* (evidenced by systemic signs of infection, tenderness and induration of the gland, and/or pus expressed from the duct in question). Depending on the degree of infection, sialadenitis due to duct obstruction can require incision and drainage or, rarely, gland excision and typically require antimicrobials.[30]

Oral Lichen Planus

Etiology

OLP is a chronic autoimmune disease that can present with a variety of symptoms and is typically more common in women in the fourth or fifth decade of life. OLP can occur by itself or in concurrence with the cutaneous form of disease as well. The cause is unknown but is proposed to be related to an immune reaction provoked by an exposure to an irritant (infections, trauma, allergens or drugs).[31] Keratinocytes undergo hydropic change followed by infiltration of mononuclear cells,[32] resulting in a precancerous lesion that may progress to squamous cell carcinoma with a frequency of 1%.[33]

Clinical presentation
Locations of the OLP lesions can be seen most commonly on the buccal mucosa and the tongue.[34] Lesions of OLP causes local discomfort, ranging from a burning sensation to severe pain, and can have the following appearances: lacelike Wickham striae (**Fig. 4**), papular, erosive (**Fig. 5**), and atrophic.[35] OLP typically appears in a symmetric distribution, most commonly on the posterior buccal mucosa.

Diagnosis
A biopsy can be used to confirm the diagnosis; however, lesions of OLP usually look like white lace-like striations along the buccal surface, red atrophic-appearing lesions, or even more erosive lesions and can be diagnosed clinically.

Treatment
Pain is the typical presenting complaint of OLP, and treatment strategies include topical or oral steroids. Steroid treatment regimens are only modestly effective, requiring high doses for courses lasting weeks or months and accompanied by their pronounced side effects, which mandate a discussion of the risks and benefits of treatment in cooperation with a primary care physician.

Aphthous Ulcer

Etiology
Also known as a canker sore, AU is the most commonly encountered oral ulcer. The condition is characterized by a painful prodrome for 2 hours to 48 hours followed by appearance of a painful round shallow ulcer that may persist for weeks.[36] No specific cause has been established, although many conditions contribute to formation of AU, including nutritional, traumatic, microbial, psychological, genetic, and allergic factors. The condition is not contagious and recurrence is the rule.

Clinical presentation
Lesions of AU appear as erythematous ulcers with a gray base and are shallow and localized (**Fig. 6**). AUs often appear as solitary lesions on the buccal or labial mucosa or on the

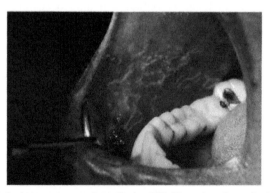

Fig. 4. Classical clinical appearance of a reticular OLP. (*From* Lauritano D, Arrica M, Lucchese A, et al. Oral lichen planus clinical characteristics in Italian patients: a retrospective analysis. Head Face Med 2016;12:18.)

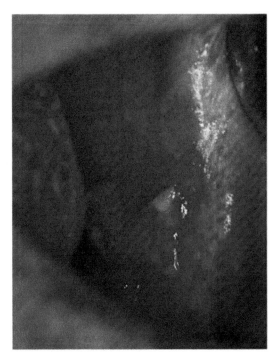

Fig. 5. Erosive OLP involving the buccal mucosa with pseudomembrane covering the erosive area. (*From* Lauritano D, Arrica M, Lucchese A, et al. Oral lichen planus clinical characteristics in Italian patients: a retrospective analysis. Head Face Med 2016;12:18.)

gingiva or tongue. Exquisite pain is typical and can affect a patient's ability to chew food in proximity to the lesion. Immunosuppressed patients (undergoing chemotherapy or human immunodeficiency virus) often have more pronounced symptoms with widespread involvement and subsequently worsening pain, which may impair oral intake.[36]

Treatment

Treatment involves relieving discomfort with protective emollients, topical anesthetic (benzocaine), topical diclofenac, or mouthwash that often includes lidocaine, Benadryl,

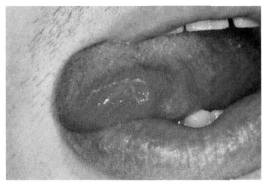

Fig. 6. Multiple aphthous ulcers on the lateral aspect of the tongue with characteristic appearance of shallow, white ulceration with surrounding erythema. (*From* Series Editor Scully C. Tongue lesions. J Investig Clin Dent. 2014;5(1):78–9; with permission.)

and antacid in combination. With more severe symptoms or extensive involvement, topical glucocorticoids can be applied to decrease AU size and duration of symptoms. Although rare, large AU ulcers may benefit from intralesional steroid injection.[36]

Oral Leukoplakia

Etiology

The term, *oral leukoplakia (OL)*, is applied to conditions presenting as white lesions of the oropharynx when other benign causes have been excluded.[37] Etiologic agents are believed to include tobacco use (smoking or chewing), alcohol consumption, betel nut chewing, and possibly infection with high-risk genotypes of human papilloma virus.[38] Rarely, or occasionally, areas of OL can evolve through dysplasia to malignancy. Areas where the mucosa is considered thinner (ventral aspect of the tongue and retromolar triangle) are subject to higher rates of transformation to carcinoma.

Clinical presentation

OL is typically a flat, whitish-color patch in the oral cavity, but the appearance can vary from a completely white and flat area, to a thick, raised white patch with red components. OL appears on the oral mucosa, gingiva, or tongue. Lesions discovered later may exhibit characteristics of malignancy, having undergone malignant transformation, although biopsy is often necessary to confirm the diagnosis.[38]

Treatment

If determined to be moderate or severe, surgical excision may be required. If only mild, OL can be treated with cryotherapy or laser ablation. Recurrence may follow if surgical margins are inadequate,[39] if smaller unrecognized areas of OL undergo malignant transformation,[40] or if the oral environment is unchanged in the postoperative period.[38]

Complications

The lesions of OL are considered premalignant. Estimating the rate of malignant transformation is difficult. Accounting for variations of follow-up and observation periods, the rate of malignant transformation of OL (often to squamous cell carcinoma) ranges between 0.13% and 17.5%, with higher established rates of transformation in patients over 50 years old.[41]

Establishing the role of risk factors (tobacco use or alcohol consumption) is less clear. Although intellectually attractive as an etiologic agent, studies attempting to establish risk of malignant transformation in tobacco use or decreased risk in tobacco cessation do not reliably demonstrate a causal relationship. Silverman and colleagues[42] demonstrated a higher risk of malignant transformation of OL in nontobacco users. A nonpremalignant form of leukoplakia is oral hairy leukoplakia, which can be caused by the Epstein-Barr virus and is almost exclusively seen in HIV-infected patients. Another form of leukoplakia that is considered rare but has a high rate of transformation to malignancy is oral proliferative verrucous leukoplakia. These lesions have a similar appearance to warts and occur more often in older women.[38] The causes for this lesion are still unknown and unrelated to the risk factors for conventional leukoplakia.

BENIGN ENTITIES

Mucocele

A mucocele is a fluid collection caused by local trauma to oral mucosa, rupturing a salivary duct and causing spillage of mucin into adjacent mucosa. Granulation tissue formation and inflammatory response may create a contained pool of mucin yielding the typical appearance of the mucocele. Local trauma is most often caused by a bite, and the distribution of mucoceles reflects this mechanism, with lower lip the most

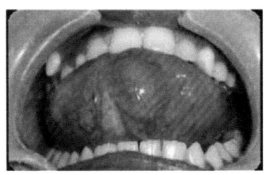

Fig. 7. Mucocele on the central inferior aspect of tongue with typical translucent or blue appearance. (*From* Khandelwal G. Micro-marsupialization: a novel non-surgical method to treat mucocele in children. J Dent Health Oral Disord Ther 2016;4(4):2; with permission.)

common location (82%).[43] Mucoceles present commonly before the fourth decade of life equally in men and women.[43]

On clinical examination (**Fig. 7**), mucoceles appear as gelatinous material and usually painless swellings that are smooth with a blue (29%), normal or pink (25%) or tan, white, or clear (18%) color.[43]

Mucoceles usually rupture spontaneously and resolve within 4 weeks to 6 weeks. If interfering with oral function, mucoceles may require surgical excision. Complete resection of the affected mucosa is necessary to avoid recurrence, and, as such, aspiration is not advised. Any patient presenting with an asymptomatic lesion not resolving after 4 weeks to 6 weeks should be advised to seek subspecialist evaluation and potential biopsy.

Bony Tori

Bony tori (**Fig. 8**) are defined as a bony protuberance that originates from the cortex of the mandible (torus mandibularis) or, more commonly, the hard palate (torus palatinus).[44] These lesions are most likely congenital but do not appear until later in life. The prevalence of bony tori is approximately 3% in the United States.[44]

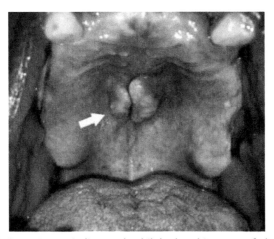

Fig. 8. Torus palatinus. Arrow indicates the bilobed architecture of the bony exostosis. (*Courtesy of* F. Madani, DMD, Philadelphia, PA; and A. Kuperstein, DDS, Philadelphia, PA.)

Tori do not cause any direct symptoms and are often incidentally noted. Occasionally, referral to an oral surgeon is required given the physical irritation or interference with the proper fit of a dental appliance or dentures. Because tori are typically painless, slow growing, and otherwise asymptomatic, the emergency provider should be alert for atypical presentations, such as masses appearing over days or weeks, associated pain or inflammation, or an evolving midline mass in the setting of an infectious process.[44]

SUMMARY

A wide array of pathologic conditions can affect the soft tissues of the mouth. The conditions typically encountered in the emergency setting can be generally organized into soft tissue and dental infections, painful but noninfectious conditions, and benign conditions that, when recognized, require little intervention. Emergency providers should be empowered with the knowledge to recognize and manage these common conditions, and through understanding, intervention, and, at times, reassurance, can improve a patient's physical and mental well-being.

REFERENCES

1. Pankhurst C. Oropharyngeal candidiasis. Clin Evid 2002;(7):1248–62.
2. Edelstein BL. The dental caries pandemic and disparities problem. BMC Oral Health 2006;6(Suppl 1):S2.
3. Klotz SA. Oropharyngeal candidiasis: a new treatment option. Clin Infect Dis 2006;42(8):1187–8.
4. Beltran-Aguilar ED, Barker LK, Canto MT, et al. Surveillance for dental caries, dental sealants, tooth retention, edentulism, and enamel fluorosis–United States, 1988-1994 and 1999-2002. MMWR Surveill Summ 2005;54(3):1–43.
5. Fontana M, Young DA, Wolff MS. Evidence-based caries, risk assessment, and treatment. Dent Clin North Am 2009;53(1):149–61, x.
6. Davies RM, Blinkhorn AS. Preventing dental caries: part 1 the scientific rationale for preventive advice. Dent Update 2013;40(9):719–20, 722,724-726.
7. Struzycka I. The oral microbiome in dental caries. Pol J Microbiol 2014;63(2): 127–35.
8. Kassebaum NJ, Bernabe E, Dahlya M, et al. Global burden of severe periodontitis in 1990-2010: a systematic review and meta-regression. J Dent Res 2014;93(11): 1045–53.
9. Wasson J, Hopkins C, Bowdler D. Did Ludwig's angina kill Ludwig? J Laryngol Otol 2006;120(5):363–5.
10. Denisco RC, Kenna GA, O'Neil MG, et al. Prevention of prescription opioid abuse: the role of the dentist. J Am Dent Assoc 2011;142(7):800–10.
11. Wertheim JO, Smith MD, Smith DM, et al. Evolutionary origins of human herpes simplex viruses 1 and 2. Mol Biol Evol 2014;31(9):2356–64.
12. Spruance SL, Nett R, Marbury T, et al. Acyclovir cream for treatment of herpes simplex labialis: results of two randomized, double-blind, vehicle-controlled, multicenter clinical trials. Antimicrob Agents Chemother 2002;46(7):2238–43.
13. Spruance SL, Stewart JC, Rowe NH, et al. Treatment of recurrent herpes simplex labialis with oral acyclovir. J Infect Dis 1990;161(2):185–90.
14. Spruance SL, Jones TM, Blatter MM, et al. High-dose, short-duration, early valacyclovir therapy for episodic treatment of cold sores: results of two randomized, placebo-controlled, multicenter studies. Antimicrob Agents Chemother 2003; 47(3):1072–80.

15. Spruance SL, Rea TL, Thoming C, et al. Penciclovir cream for the treatment of herpes simplex labialis. A randomized, multicenter, double-blind, placebo-controlled trial. Topical Penciclovir Collaborative Study Group. JAMA 1997; 277(17):1374–9.
16. Cunningham A, Griffiths P, Leone P, et al. Current management and recommendations for access to antiviral therapy of herpes labialis. J Clin Virol 2012;53(1): 6–11.
17. Leung AKC, Barankin B. Herpes labialis: an update. Recent Pat Inflamm Allergy Drug Discov 2017;11(2):107–13.
18. Rooney JF, Straus SE, Mannix ML, et al. Oral acyclovir to suppress frequently recurrent herpes labialis. A double-blind, placebo-controlled trial. Ann Intern Med 1993;118(4):268–72.
19. Worrall G. Acyclovir in recurrent herpes labialis. BMJ 1996;312(7022):6.
20. Arduino PG, Porter SR. Oral and perioral herpes simplex virus type 1 (HSV-1) infection: review of its management. Oral Dis 2006;12(3):254–70.
21. Gilbert SC. Management and prevention of recurrent herpes labialis in immunocompetent patients. Herpes 2007;14(3):56–61.
22. Chentoufi AA, Zhang X, Lamberth K, et al. HLA-A*0201-restricted CD8+ cytotoxic T lymphocyte epitopes identified from herpes simplex virus glycoprotein D. J Immunol 2008;180(1):426–37.
23. Kim M, Taylor J, Sidney J, et al. Immunodominant epitopes in herpes simplex virus type 2 glycoprotein D are recognized by CD4 lymphocytes from both HSV-1 and HSV-2 seropositive subjects. J Immunol 2008;181(9):6604–15.
24. Dropulic LK, Cohen JI. The challenge of developing a herpes simplex virus 2 vaccine. Expert Rev Vaccines 2012;11(12):1429–40.
25. Ramanojam S, Merchant Y, Bhardwaj S, et al. Idiopathic sialolithiasis: scalpel versus current trends in management. J Craniofac Surg 2017;28(4):e363–4.
26. Ellies M, Laskawi R, Arglebe C, et al. Surgical management of nonneoplastic diseases of the submandibular gland: a follow-up study. Int J Oral Maxillofac Surg 1996;25(4):285–9.
27. Afzelius P, Nielsen M-Y, Ewertsen C, et al. Imaging of the major salivary glands. Clin Physiol Funct Imaging 2016;36(1):1–10.
28. Evirgen S, Kamburoglu K. Review on the applications of ultrasonography in dentomaxillofacial region. World J Radiol 2016;8(1):50–8.
29. Brown JE, Escudier MP, Whaites EJ, et al. Intra-oral ultrasound imaging of a submandibular duct calculus. Dentomaxillofac Radiol 1997;26(4):252–5.
30. Armstrong MA, Turturro MA. Salivary gland emergencies. Emerg Med Clin North Am 2013;31(2):481–99.
31. Wagner G, Rose C, Sachse M. Clinical variants of lichen planus. J Dtsch Dermatol Ges 2013;11(4):309–19.
32. Nosratzehi T. Oral lichen planus: an overview of potential risk factors, biomarkers and treatments. Asian Pac J Cancer Prev 2018;19(5):1161–7.
33. Lauritano D, Arrica M, Lucchese A, et al. Oral lichen planus clinical characteristics in Italian patients: a retrospective analysis. Head Face Med 2016;12:18.
34. Rivera C, Jones-Herrera C, Vargas P. Oral diseases- a 14 year experience of a Chilean institution with a systematic review from eight countries. Med Oral Patol Oral Cir Bucal 2017;22(3):e297–306.
35. Le Cleach L, Chosidow O. Clinical practice: lichen planus. N Engl J Med 2012; 366(8):723–32.
36. Akintoye SO, Greenberg MS. Recurrent aphthous stomatitis. Dent Clin North Am 2014;58(2):281–7.

37. Arduino PG, Bagan J, El-Naggar AK, et al. Urban legends series: oral leukoplakia. Oral Dis 2013;19(7):642–59.
38. Amagasa T, Yamashiro M, Uzawa N. Oral premalignant lesions: from a clinical perspective. Int J Clin Oncol 2011;16(1):5–14.
39. van der Waal I, Schepman KP, van der Meij EH, et al. Oral leukoplakia: a clinicopathological review. Oral Oncol 1997;33(5):291–301.
40. Scholes AG, Woolgar JA, Boyle MA, et al. Synchronous oral carcinomas: independent or common clonal origin? Cancer Res 1998;58(9):2003–6.
41. Amagasa T, Yamashiro M, Ishikawa H. Oral leukoplakia related to malignant transformation. Oral Sci Int 2006;3:45–55.
42. Silverman JS, Meir G, Ms Francina Lozada D. Oral leukoplakia and malignant transformation. A follow-up study of 257 patients. Cancer 2018;53(3):563–8.
43. Chi AC, Lambert PR 3rd, Richardson MS, et al. Oral mucoceles: a clinicopathologic review of 1,824 cases, including unusual variants. J Oral Maxillofac Surg 2011;69(4):1086–93.
44. Madani FM, Kuperstein AS. Normal variations of oral anatomy and common oral soft tissue lesions: evaluation and management. Med Clin North Am 2014;98(6):1281–98.
45. Selwitz RH, Ismail AI, Pitts NB. Dental caries. Lancet 2007;369(9555):51–9.
46. Abernathy JR, Graves RC, Greenberg BG, et al. Application of life table methodology in determining dental caries rates. Community Dent Oral Epidemiol 1986;14(5):261–4.
47. Mejare I, Stenlund H, Zelezny-Holmlund C. Caries incidence and lesion progression from adolescence to young adulthood: a prospective 15-year cohort study in Sweden. Caries Res 2004;38(2):130–41.
48. Carlos JP, Gittelsohn AM. Longitudinal studies of the natural history of caries. I. Eruption patterns of the permanent teeth. J Dent Res 1965;44:509–16.
49. Ismail AI, Lim S, Sohn W, et al. Determinants of early childhood caries in low-income African American young children. Pediatr Dent 2008;30(4):289–96.

Infections of the Oropharynx

Matthew R. Klein, MD, MPH

KEYWORDS

- Streptococcal pharyngitis • Infectious mononucleosis • Peritonsillar abscess
- Retropharyngeal abscess • Epiglottitis

KEY POINTS

- Oropharyngeal infections include a broad spectrum of severity from mild illness to complete airway obstruction.
- Emergency clinicians should anticipate the need for a surgical airway in patients with signs of airway obstruction.
- A clinical decision tool, in conjunction with rapid antigen detection tests, can help identify patients with group A beta-hemolytic strep pharyngitis.
- A mononucleosis heterophile antibody test may be negative in 25% of patients during the first week of illness and in 5% to 10% of patients in the second week and beyond.
- Because of the vaccination against *Haemophilus influenzae* type B, epiglottitis is now more common in adults than children.

INTRODUCTION

The chief complaint of "sore throat" is commonly encountered in the emergency department (ED) and requires clinicians to answer the fundamental question of emergency medicine: Is this patient "sick" or "not sick"? The oropharynx extends from the soft palate to the hyoid bone, and infections in this anatomic space range from mild self-limited illness, to airway compromise, sepsis, and death. Emergency clinicians must maintain a high index of suspicion when evaluating patients with oropharyngeal infections and consider a broad differential diagnosis. This article reviews the presentation, diagnosis, and management of common and "can't miss" infections of the oropharynx, including streptococcal pharyngitis, infectious mononucleosis (IM), peritonsillar abscess (PTA), retropharyngeal abscess (RPA), and epiglottitis.

Disclosure Statement: The author has no financial interests to disclose.
Department of Emergency Medicine, Northwestern University, 211 East Ontario – Suite 300, Chicago, IL 60611, USA
E-mail address: Matthew.richard.klein@gmail.com

Emerg Med Clin N Am 37 (2019) 69–80
https://doi.org/10.1016/j.emc.2018.09.002　　　　　　　　　　**emed.theclinics.com**
0733-8627/19/© 2018 Elsevier Inc. All rights reserved.

INITIAL EMERGENCY DEPARTMENT EVALUATION

Patients with suspected oropharyngeal infections should be promptly evaluated for signs of airway compromise (**Box 1**). If present, empiric antibiotics and steroids should be administered. Airway management may be required. In cases of severe obstruction, a surgical airway may be necessary, in conjunction with otolaryngology consultation, if available. Patients with oropharyngeal infections can be dehydrated due to decreased oral intake or insensible losses and may require fluid resuscitation. In the absence of airway compromise, management should proceed based on the likely diagnosis. Important historical factors to ascertain include time course of symptoms, immune status, and allergies to antibiotics.

STREPTOCOCCAL PHARYNGITIS

With "sore throat" accounting for 1% to 2% of all ambulatory health care visits in the United States, distinguishing group A beta-hemolytic streptococcus (GAS) from viral pharyngitis is a common clinical scenario for emergency clinicians.[1] Differentiating between viral and bacterial pharyngitis is difficult because of nonspecific and overlapping symptoms, particularly among younger patients, who may be more likely to present with coryza, nausea, and vomiting, and less likely to present with exudates than adults.[2] Nevertheless, making an accurate diagnosis is important, because GAS infection can lead to suppurative (sinusitis, acute otitis media, PTA) and nonsuppurative (glomerulonephritis, rheumatic fever) complications.[3]

Cause

Throat culture isolates are positive for GAS in 5% to 24% of adults and 24% to 36% of children with a sore throat.[4] Peak incidence of GAS pharyngitis occurs between ages 5 and 10 years, and it is more common during late winter and early spring.[5]

Diagnosis

Because of its nonspecific signs and symptoms, diagnosing GAS pharyngitis based on history and physical examination alone can be challenging. The modified Centor (also known as McIssac) score is commonly used when considering whom to test and treat for GAS and has been validated in children and adults.[6] **Table 1** lists the modified Centor criteria, and the risk of GAS pharyngitis based on Centor score is presented in **Table 2**.

For patients with a modified Centor score of zero or less, there is general consensus that no additional testing or treatment is necessary. In patients with a modified Centor score greater than zero, recommendations to perform a rapid antigen detection test (RADT) or treat empirically differ by specialty society, particularly for a score of 3 and 4.[3,7] The Infectious Disease Society of America does not recommend testing

---

Box 1
Signs of airway compromise

Sniffing position (sitting upright with neck extended)

Drooling

Muffled voice

Stridor

Hypoxia

Table 1
Modified Centor criteria

Criteria	Points
Absence of cough	+1
Swollen, tender anterior cervical lymph nodes	+1
Temperature >38°C (100.4°F)	+1
Tonsillar exudates or swelling	+1
Age 3–14 y	+1
Age 15–44 y	0
45 y or older	−1

Adapted from McIsaac WJ, White D, Tannenbaum D, et al. A clinical score to reduce unnecessary antibiotic use in patients with sore throat. CMAJ 1998;158(1):79; with permission.

for GAS pharyngitis or empirically treating in children younger than 3 years of age in the absence of other risk factors like an older sibling with GAS, due to the low prevalence of disease in this age group.[8]

In children, RADT scores are 85% to 87% sensitive and 95% to 96% specific; in adults, sensitivity ranges from 87% to 94% and specificity ranges from 92% to 95%.[9] Throat cultures may be obtained, particularly in patients with a negative RADT, but results will not be available during the initial ED visit.

Management

GAS is a self-limited disease and typically resolves after several days, even in the absence of treatment. Antibiotics can reduce the length of symptoms by 16 hours and are frequently prescribed with the goal of reducing suppurative complications from GAS.[10] Nonsuppurative complications may also be prevented by antibiotics; however, these are uncommon in high-income countries.[11]

A single dose of 1.2 million units (or 600,000 units if <27 kg) intramuscular benzathine penicillin G or a 10-day course of oral penicillin or amoxicillin is recommended for treatment of GAS pharyngitis. Clindamycin, azithromycin, or a cephalosporin may be used in patients with a penicillin allergy.[12] Children may return to school after 24 hours of antibiotic treatment.

A systematic review and meta-analysis found that a single dose of corticosteroids can provide pain relief in patients with sore throat, without an increase in serious adverse events.[13] Acetaminophen and ibuprofen may also be used for analgesia.

INFECTIOUS MONONUCLEOSIS

Alternately referred to as "glandular fever" or the "kissing disease," IM classically presents as a sore throat with associated fever and lymphadenopathy and is most

Table 2
Risk of group A beta-hemolytic streptococcus pharyngitis based on Centor score

Modified Centor Score	Risk of GAS Pharyngitis, %
≥4	51–53
3	28–35
2	11–17
1	5–10
≤0	1–2.5

commonly encountered in patients aged 15 to 24 years.[14] Because of its nonspecific symptoms, IM easily mimics bacterial and viral pharyngitis, although symptoms of IM (particularly fatigue) may persist for weeks to several months.

Cause

IM is most commonly caused by Epstein-Barr virus (EBV), which infects 95% of the world's population and is transmitted through infected saliva, primarily during childhood or adolescence.[15] When entertaining the possibility of IM, emergency clinicians should also consider screening for human immunodeficiency virus in at-risk patients, as well as cytomegalovirus and toxoplasmosis, particularly in pregnant women.

Diagnosis

Symptoms of IM, including sore throat, fatigue, and headache, are nonspecific, making it challenging to differentiate IM from other viral syndromes.[16] **Table 3** lists likelihood ratios (LRs) for clinical findings associated with IM.[17]

Emergency clinicians should be aware of the limitations of heterophile antibody (mononucleosis spot) testing, which, as with all diagnostics, must be interpreted in the context of a patient's symptoms.[18] Heterophile antibody testing is 85% sensitive and 94% specific for IM and is negative in 25% of patients with IM during the first week of illness, and in 5% to 10% of patients in the second week and beyond.[15]

Management

Treatment of IM is primarily supportive care, with antipyretics and anti-inflammatories provided for symptom relief. Antiviral medications have not been shown to yield clinically significant benefits. A 2015 Cochrane Review found insufficient evidence for steroid use in treating symptoms of IM.[19]

Several complications can result from IM. Neurologic sequelae include meningoencephalitis, optic neuritis, facial nerve palsy, transverse myelitis, and Guillain-Barré syndrome.[20] Hemolytic anemia, thrombocytopenia, and agranulocytosis may also occur after EBV infection.[21] Rarely, airway obstruction can result from palatal and nasopharyngeal tonsillar hypertrophy, particularly in children.[22]

Male patients under the age of 30 years within 4 weeks of onset of IM symptoms appear to be at highest risk for splenic rupture, which may occur without trauma.[23] However, splenic rupture has been reported up to 8 weeks after developing infectious symptoms, and patients with IM should be counseled to avoid physical activity for 1 to 2 months.[24] Serial splenic ultrasound may allow for a more rapid return to contact sports.[25]

Table 3 Clinical findings that suggest infectious mononucleosis		
Clinical Finding	Positive LR	Negative LR
Atypical lymphocytes ≥10%	11	0.37
Palatine petechiae	5.3	1.0
Splenomegaly	1.9–6.6	0.65–0.94
Posterior cervical lymphadenopathy	3.1	0.69
Inguinal or axillary lymphadenopathy (or both)	3.0–3.3	0.57–0.81

PERITONSILLAR ABSCESS

Historically known as "quinsy," PTAs form in the space between the palatine tonsil and its capsule and typically present with the following signs and symptoms[26]:

- Fever
- Malaise
- Trismus
- Drooling
- Muffled voice

Unilateral swelling and contralateral displacement of the uvula is classic; however, rare cases of bilateral PTAs with a midline uvula have been reported.[27] Uncommonly, an aberrant internal carotid artery can result in unilateral swelling of the peritonsillar space and mimic the presentation of a PTA.[28,29] Complications of a PTA include airway obstruction, abscess rupture and aspiration, hemorrhage from erosion into the carotid sheath, and extension into deep spaces of the neck and mediastinum.[30]

Cause

A PTA can result from progression of tonsillar inflammation, tonsillar cellulitis, and obstruction of salivary glands located in the soft palate known as Weber glands. Abscess isolates are frequently polymicrobial, with both aerobic and anaerobic organisms. Common bacteria include *Streptococcus pyogenes*, *Staphylococcus aureus*, *Haemophilus influenzae*, as well as *Prevotella*, *Porphyromonas*, *Fusobacterium*, and *Peptostreptococcus* species.[31]

Diagnosis

Although PTA can be diagnosed based on physical examination alone, clinical impression is only 78% sensitive and 50% specific.[32] Computed tomography (CT) is superior to clinical impression, with 100% sensitivity and 75% specificity, but is associated with increased cost and radiation exposure for the patient.[32] Intraoral or transcutaneous point-of-care ultrasound (POCUS) examinations can also identify PTA.[33,34] Using POCUS for PTA drainage has been shown to decrease patient cost and need for otolaryngology consultation.[35] However, use of POCUS may be limited by equipment availability, and variation in performance characteristics exist depending on operator skill.

Management

Surgical management of PTA involves one of 3 approaches: tonsillectomy, incision and drainage (I&D), and needle aspiration.[36] Both tonsillectomy and I&D typically require otolaryngology consultation. A systematic review of I&D versus needle aspiration found very low-quality evidence to suggest I&D may be associated with lower recurrence, and that needle aspiration may be less painful for patients.[37] Needle aspiration is commonly used by emergency clinicians. Local or topical anesthesia should be provided. An 18-gauge needle attached to a 10-mL syringe can be used for aspiration. Care should be taken to avoid the internal carotid artery. To prevent inserting the needle too deeply, the distal 1 cm of the plastic needle guard can be cut off, and the guard reattached to the syringe over the needle. A laryngoscope, or the bottom half of a disposable plastic speculum with a light source, can be placed into the mouth with the patient sitting up to help control the patient's tongue and provide sufficient illumination (**Fig. 1**).[38]

Although data are limited, administration of intravenous (IV) steroids seems to result in reduced pain and may prompt faster recovery, without report of adverse side

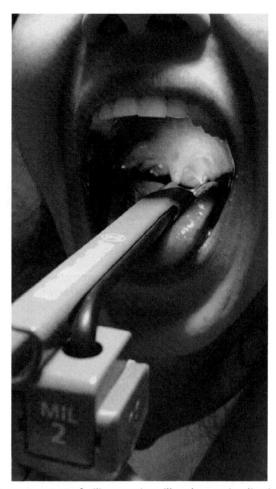

Fig. 1. Use of a laryngoscope to facilitate peritonsillar abscess visualization.

effects.[39,40] Both dexamethasone 8 to 10 mg IV and methylprednisolone 2 to 3 mg/kg IV have been studied.

Empiric antibiotics should be provided and should cover *Streptococcus* and *Staphylococcus* species as well as anaerobes. Common regimens include clindamycin, amoxicillin/clavulanate, or ampicillin/sulbactam.[36]

Well-appearing patients without airway compromise who can tolerate oral intake may be candidates for discharge from the ED. However, patients with systemic signs of infection, need for continued airway monitoring, or inability to tolerate oral intake require admission to an observation or inpatient setting.

RETROPHARYNGEAL ABSCESS

Infections of the retropharyngeal space, a potential space that extends from the base of the skull to the posterior mediastinum, can lead to devastating complications, including airway obstruction, vascular compromise, mediastinitis, and vertebral osteomyelitis.[41] RPA is more frequently seen in children than adults, particularly those younger than 5 years, and there is a higher incidence in boys and men. Although RPA is uncommon, data from a large registry of patients younger than 20 years showed increasing incidence from 2.98 per 100,000 in 2003 to 4.10 per 100,000 in 2012.[42]

Clinical features concerning for RPA include the following[43]:

- Fever
- Neck pain/swelling
- Cervical lymphadenopathy
- Nuchal rigidity or torticollis
- Drooling
- Stridor

Cause

RPAs are thought to result from extension of nasopharyngeal infections to retropharyngeal lymph nodes.[44] These lymph nodes atrophy by the time of puberty, which helps explain why RPA is less commonly seen in adults. RPA may also occur as a result of local trauma from objects like fish or chicken bones.[45] Similar to PTA, RPA isolates are commonly polymicrobial, with group A beta-hemolytic streptococci, *S aureus*, *Fusobacterium*, *Bacteroides*, and *Prevotella* species identified as causative bacteria.[31]

Diagnosis

Lateral soft tissue neck radiographs may be used as an initial screening test for RPA and should be performed during inspiration with the neck in extension.[46] The presence of gas or air-fluid levels in the soft tissue, and widening of the prevertebral space beyond 5 to 7 mm at the level of the second cervical vertebrae, or 14 mm in a child (22 mm in an adult) at the level of the sixth cervical vertebrae, should raise suspicion for RPA.[47,48]

Compared with plain radiography, CT and MRI are better able to distinguish RPA from other entities, such as retropharyngeal edema or a suppurative retropharyngeal node.[49] In one series of patients with retropharyngeal or parapharyngeal infections, intraoperative findings confirmed CT interpretation in 76.3% of cases, with false-positive and false-negative rates of 13.2% and 10.5%, respectively.[50] Discordance between CT and operative findings has been reported in other case series, suggesting that although CT remains helpful in the diagnosis of RPA, surgical exploration remains the gold standard.[51,52]

Management

Patients with RPA who present with respiratory distress must be considered at risk for imminent airway obstruction and require immediate airway management. When available, an otolaryngologist should be consulted because these patients may require a surgical airway and operative drainage. IV steroids and empiric antibiotics with gram-positive and anaerobic coverage (such as clindamycin, ampicillin/sulbactam, or amoxicillin/clavulanate) should be administered promptly.

In stable patients, debate exists over surgical or conservative management of RPA, and high-quality evidence is lacking. Factors that should prompt surgical drainage include airway compromise, sepsis, and lack of improvement after 48 hours of IV antibiotic therapy.[53] In one retrospective review of 54 pediatric patients with RPA or PTA identified on cross-sectional imaging, a majority (70%) were treated with antibiotics alone for at least 24 hours. In this cohort, younger patients with abscess diameter less than 25 mm were more likely to require surgical drainage than older children.[54] A separate series of 178 pediatric patients with RPA or PTA also found an increased need for surgical drainage in children younger than 15 months with abscess diameter greater than 22 mm.[55]

EPIGLOTTITIS

Cited as a possible culprit in the death of George Washington, epiglottitis, also known as supraglottitis, refers to inflammation of the epiglottis and surrounding structures, which places patients at risk for airway obstruction.[56] Epiglottitis due to *Haemophilus influenzae* type B (Hib) was previously seen primarily in children; however, since the adoption of widespread vaccination against Hib, it is evolving into a disease of adults.[57] From 1995 to 2006, incidence decreased in the United States, with a mean age of 45 years.[58]

Symptoms of epiglottitis include the following[59]:

- Odynophagia/dysphagia
- Voice change
- Tachycardia
- Drooling
- Fever
- Tachypnea
- Stridor
- Respiratory distress

Cause

The success of the Hib vaccine resulted in a 95% reduction in Hib-related disease, which significantly altered the microbiology of epiglottitis.[60] Although cases of vaccine failure still occur, *Streptococcus pneumoniae* and *S aureus*, in addition to *Moraxella*, *Pseudomonas*, and *Neisseria* species, are now more common causes of epiglottitis than in the prevaccine era.[61]

Diagnosis

Emergency clinicians must maintain a high index of suspicion for epiglottitis in both children and adults, particularly those who appear toxic with signs of airway obstruction. Lateral soft tissue neck radiographs may reveal a "thumblike" epiglottis, and an epiglottis width of greater than 6.3 mm is 97.8% specific for acute epiglottitis.[46,62] Presence of an "alphabet P sign" on bedside ultrasound may also aid in the diagnosis.[63] In one patient series, elevated C-reactive protein, hyperglycemia, and relative neutrophilia were associated with airway intervention and admission to an intensive care unit (ICU).[64] Visualization of the epiglottis, whether by direct laryngoscopy, nasopharyngoscopy, or bronchoscopy, remains the gold standard for diagnosis.[65]

Management

Similar to other oropharyngeal infections, management of acute epiglottitis requires airway assessment, prompt administration of IV antibiotics, and hospital admission, commonly to an ICU. The use of corticosteroids remains controversial, and high-quality data are lacking.[65,66] Despite the appropriate concern for airway obstruction, the overall rate of intubation in patients with epiglottitis remains low. In a retrospective analysis of pediatric and adult epiglottitis patients using data from the National Inpatient Sample, 16% of patients required intubation and 3% underwent tracheotomy.[58] A separate series of 342 pediatric patients with acute epiglottitis identified 40 cases (11%) that required intubation or tracheotomy.[67]

SUMMARY

Oropharyngeal infections include a spectrum of diseases ranging from mild, self-limited illness to acute life threats requiring immediate airway management. Emergency clinicians should perform a prompt airway assessment on all patients presenting with a complaint of "sore throat" and remain vigilant for signs of airway compromise. Careful attention to key historical and physical examination features can narrow a broad differential diagnosis and guide appropriate treatment.

REFERENCES

1. Alcaide M, Bisno A. Pharyngitis and epiglottitis. Infect Dis Clin North Am 2007; 21(2):449–69.
2. Wessels M. Clinical practice. Streptococcal pharyngitis. N Engl J Med 2011; 364(7):648–55.
3. Gottlieb M, Long B, Koyfman A. Clinical mimics: an emergency medicine-focused review of streptococcal pharyngitis mimics. J Emerg Med 2018;54(5): 619–29.
4. Ebell M, Smith M, Barry H, et al. The rational clinical examination. Does this patient have strep throat? JAMA 2000;284(22):2912–8.
5. Kalra M, Higgins K, Perez E. Common questions about streptococcal pharyngitis. Am Fam Physician 2016;94(1):24–31.
6. McIssac W, Goel V, To T, et al. The validity of a sore throat score in family practice. CMAJ 2000;163(7):811–5.
7. Matthys J, De Meyere M, van Driel M, et al. Differences among international pharyngitis guidelines: not just academic. Ann Fam Med 2007;5(5):436–43.
8. Shulman S, Bisno A, Clegg H, et al. Clinical practice guideline for the diagnosis and management of group A streptococcal pharyngitis: 2012 update by the Infectious Diseases Society of America. Clin Infect Dis 2012;55(10):1279–82.
9. Stewart E, Davis B, Clemans-Taylor B, et al. Rapid antigen group A streptococcus test to diagnose pharyngitis: a systematic review and meta-analysis. PLoS One 2014;9(11):e111727.
10. Choby B. Diagnosis and treatment of streptococcal pharyngitis. Am Fam Physician 2009;79(5):383–90.
11. Spinka A, Glaszious P, Del Mar C. Antibiotics for sore throat. Cochrane Database Syst Rev 2013;(11):CD000023.
12. Randel A. IDSA updates guidelines for managing group A streptococcal pharyngitis. Am Fam Physician 2013;88(5):338–40.
13. Sadeghirad B, Siemieniuk R, Brignardello-Petersen R, et al. Corticosteroids for treatment of sore throat: systematic review and meta-analysis of randomised trials. BMJ 2017;358:j3887.
14. Womack J, Jimenez M. Common questions about infectious mononucleosis. Am Fam Physician 2015;91(6):372–6.
15. Luzuriaga K, Sullivan J. Infectious mononucleosis. N Engl J Med 2010;362(21): 1993–2000.
16. Ebell M, Call M, Shinholser J, et al. Does this patient have infectious mononucleosis?: the rational clinical examination systematic review. JAMA 2016;315(14): 1502–9.
17. Welch J, Holland D. What elements suggest infectious mononucleosis? Ann Emerg Med 2018;71(4):521–2.
18. Jordan M, Englof I, Rix R, et al. Mononucleosis testing in the emergency department: correlation with signs and symptoms. Ann Emerg Med 2013;62(4):S152–3.

19. Rezek E, Nofal Y, Hamzeh A, et al. Steroids for symptom control in infectious mononucleosis. Cochrane Database Syst Rev 2015;(11):CD004402.
20. Jenson H. Acute complications of Epstein-Barr virus infectious mononucleosis. Curr Opin Pediatr 2000;12(3):263–8.
21. Massoll A, Powers S, Betten D. Agranulocytosis occurrence following recent acute infectious mononucleosis. Am J Emerg Med 2017;35(5):803.e5-6.
22. Wohl D, Isaacson J. Airway obstruction in children with infectious mononucleosis. Ear Nose Throat J 1995;74(9):630–8.
23. Bartlett A, Williams R, Hilton M. Splenic rupture in infectious mononucleosis: a systematic review of published case reports. Injury 2016;47:531.
24. Shephard R. Exercise and the athlete with infectious mononucleosis. Clin J Sport Med 2017;27(2):168–78.
25. O'Connor T, SKinner L, Kiely P, et al. Return to contact sports following infectious mononucleosis: the role of serial ultrasonography. Ear Nose Throat J 2011;90(8): E21-4.
26. Galioto N. Peritonsillar abscess. Am Fam Physician 2008;77:199–202.
27. Fasano CJ, Chudnofsky C, Vanderbeek P. Bilateral peritonsillar abscesses: not your usual sore throat. J Emerg Med 2005;29(1):45–7.
28. Lo CC, Luo CM, Fang TJ. Aberrant internal carotid artery in the mouth mimicking peritonsillar abscess. Am J Emerg Med 2010;28(2):259.e5-6.
29. Tsunoda K, Takanosawa M, Matsuda K. Aberrant internal carotid artery in the mouth. Lancet 1997;250(9074):340.
30. Powell J, Wilson JA. An evidence-based review of peritonsillar abscess. Clin Otolaryngol 2012;37:136–45.
31. Brook I. Microbiology and management of peritonsillar, retropharyngeal, and parapharyngeal abscesses. J Oral Maxillofac Surg 2004;62:1545–50.
32. Scott PM, Loftus WK, Kew J, et al. Diagnosis of peritonsillar infections: a prospective study of ultrasound, computerized tomography and clinical diagnosis. J Laryngol Otol 1999;113(3):229–32.
33. Secko M, Sivitz A. Think ultrasound first for peritonsillar swelling. Am J Emerg Med 2015;33(4):569–72.
34. Nogan S, Jandali D, Cipolla M, et al. The use of ultrasound imaging in evaluation of peritonsillar infections. Laryngoscope 2015;125(11):2604–7.
35. Froehlich M, Huang Z, Reilly R. Utilization of ultrasound for diagnostic evaluation and management of peritonsillar abscess. Curr Opin Otolaryngol Head Neck Surg 2017;25:163–8.
36. Herzon F, Martin A. Medical and surgical treatment of peritonsillar, retropharyngeal, and parapharyngeal abscesses. Curr Infect Dis Rep 2006;8:196–202.
37. Chang B, Thamboo A, Burton MJ, et al. Needle aspiration versus incision and drainage for the treatment of peritonsillar abscess. Cochrane Database Syst Rev 2016;(12):CD006287.
38. Brode DA, Shalit M. A novel approach to enhance visualization during drainage of peritonsillar abscess. J Emerg Med 2008;35(3):297–8.
39. Chau JK, Seikaly HR, Harris JR, et al. Corticosteroids in peritonsillar abscess treatment: a blinded placebo-controlled clinical trial. Laryngoscope 2014;124: 97–103.
40. Hurr K, Zhou S, Kysh L. Adjunct steroids in the treatment of peritonsillar abscess: a systematic review. Laryngoscope 2018;128:72–7.
41. Jang YJ, Rhee CK. Retropharyngeal abscess associated with vertebral osteomyelitis and spinal epidural sabscess. Otolaryngol Head Neck Surg 1998;119(6): 705–8.

42. Woods CR, Cash ED, Smith AM, et al. Retropharyngeal and parapharyngeal abscesses among children and adolescents in the United States: epidemiology and management trends, 2003-2012. J Pediatric Infect Dis Soc 2016;5(3):258–68.
43. Gaglani MJ, Edwards MS. Clinical indicators of childhood retropharyngeal abscess. Am J Emerg Med 1995;13(3):333–6.
44. Craig FW, Schunk JE. Retropharyngeal abscess in children: clinical presentation, utility of imaging, and current management. Pediatrics 2003;111(6 Pt 1):1394–8.
45. Poluri A, Singh B, Sperlin N, et al. Retropharyngeal abscess secondary to penetrating foreign bodies. J Craniomaxillofac Surg 2000;28(4):243–6.
46. Virk JS, Pang J, Okhovat S, et al. Analysing lateral soft tissue neck radiographs. Emerg Radiol 2012;19(3):255–60.
47. McLeod C, Stanley KA. Imagines in emergency medicine: retropharyngeal abscess. West J Emerg Med 2008;9(1):55.
48. Brechtelsbauer PB, Garetz SL, Gebarski SS, et al. Retropharyngeal abscess: pitfalls of plain films and computed tomography. Am J Otolaryngol 1997;18(4): 258–62.
49. Hoang JK, Branstetter BF, Eastwood JD, et al. Multiplanar CT and MRI of collections in the retropharyngeal space: is it an abscess? Am J Roentgenol 2011; 196(4):W426–32.
50. Lazor JB, Cunningham MJ, Eavey RD, et al. Comparison of computed tomography and surgical findings in deep neck infections. Otolaryngol Head Neck Surg 1994;111(6):746–50.
51. Grisaru-Soen G, Komisar O, Aizenstein O, et al. Retropharyngeal and parapharyngeal abscess in children - epidemiology, clinical features and treatment. Int J Pediatr Otorhinolaryngol 2010;74(9):1016–20.
52. Daya H, Lo S, Papsin BC, et al. Retropharyngeal and parapharyngeal infections in children: the Toronto experience. Int J Pediatr Otorhinolaryngol 2005;69(1): 81–6.
53. Lawrence R, Bateman N. Controversies in the management of deep neck space infection in children: an evidence-based review. Clin Otolaryngol 2017;42(1): 156–63.
54. Wong DK, Brown C, Mills N, et al. To drain or not to drain - management of pediatric deep neck abscesses: a case-control study. Int J Pediatr Otorhinolaryngol 2012;76(12):1810–3.
55. Chen J, Elden L. Children with deep space neck infections: our experience with 178 children. Otolaryngol Head Neck Surg 2013;148(6):1037–42.
56. Morens D. Death of a president. N Engl J Med 1999;341(24):1845–9.
57. Guldfred LA, Lyhne D, Becker B. Acute epiglottitis: epidemiology, clinical presentation, management and outcome. J Laryngol Otol 2008;122(8):818–23.
58. Shah R, Stocks C. Epiglottitis in the United States: national trends, variances, prognosis, and management. Laryngoscope 2010;120(6):1256–62.
59. Guardiani E, Bliss M, Harley E. Supraglottitis in the era following widespread immunization against Haemophilus influenzae type B: evolving principes in diagnosis and management. Laryngoscope 2010;120(11):2183–8.
60. Wenger D. Epidemiology of Haemophilus influenzae type b disease and impact of Haemophilus influenzae type b conjugate vaccines in the United States and Canada. Pediatr Infect Dis J 1998;17(9 Suppl):S132–6.
61. Shah R, Roberson D, Jones D. Epiglottitis in the Hemophilus influenzae type B vaccine era: changing trends. Laryngoscope 2004;114(3):557–60.
62. Lee S, Yun S, Kim D, et al. Do we need a change in ED diagnostic strategy for adult acute epiglottitis? Am J Emerg Med 2017;35(10):1519–24.

63. Hung T, Li S, Chen P, et al. Bedside ultrasonography as a safe and effective tool to diagnose acute epiglottitis. Am J Emerg Med 2011;29(3):359.e1-3.
64. Galitz Y, Shoffel-Havakuk H, Cohen O, et al. Adult acute supraglottitis: analysis of 358 patients for predictors of airway intervention. Laryngoscope 2017;127(9): 2106–12.
65. Glynn F, Fenton J. Diagnosis and management of supraglottitis (epiglottitis). Curr Infect Dis Rep 2008;10(3):200–4.
66. Phillips J, Innes A, Naik M. Corticosteroids for supraglottitis. Br J Anaesth 2004; 92(3):454–5.
67. Acevedo J, Lander L, Choi S, et al. Airway management in pediatric epiglottitis: a national perspective. Otolaryngol Head Neck Surg 2009;140(4):548–51.

Dental Emergencies

Jean M. Hammel, MD*, Jason Fischel, MD, MPH

KEYWORDS

- Dental fractures • Dental infections • Dental blocks • Tooth avulsion and luxation

KEY POINTS

- The anatomy of the mouth, including the eruption sequence of primary teeth, is important in diagnosing and treating dental emergencies.
- With traumatic fractures, loosening, or complete avulsion of the tooth, the primary goal of treatment is to preserve or restore the integrity of the tooth and the secondary goal is cosmesis.
- Primary teeth are never replaced if avulsed.
- Dental infections range from simple caries to life-threatening infections, such as acute necrotizing ulcerative gingivitis and Ludwig angina. In the emergency department (ED), assessing the extent of infection, antibiotic and analgesia administration, imaging, and prompt referral to a dentist or oral surgeon are paramount.
- Key ED procedures include dental blocks for pain relief, reducing and splinting teeth, and achieving hemostasis.

INTRODUCTION AND EPIDEMIOLOGY

Dental emergencies are common problems seen in the emergency department (ED). Approximately 750,000 visits are made to EDs annually for dental problems.[1,2] Pain, trauma, and infection are 3 of the most frequent complaints. For the most part, dental emergencies are not life-threatening but can be painful and/or cosmetically significant. A disproportionate number of patients may come to the ED due to lack of access to a primary dentist and/or dental insurance.[3,4] However, a significant number of patients with acute dental trauma cannot wait for business hours due to associated pain, bleeding, or concomitant injuries. Therefore, emergency physicians must be well-versed in the evaluation and management of these issues.

ANATOMY

The approach to assessing dental injuries and discomfort begins with an understanding of oral anatomy and development. The tooth itself comprises the outer layer of

Disclosure Statement: No disclosures to report.
Department of Emergency Medicine, Norwalk Hospital, 34 Maple Street, Norwalk, CT 06850, USA
* Corresponding author.
E-mail address: Jean.hammel@wchn.org

Emerg Med Clin N Am 37 (2019) 81–93
https://doi.org/10.1016/j.emc.2018.09.008
0733-8627/19/© 2018 Elsevier Inc. All rights reserved.

enamel, an inner layer of dentin, and the inner structure of pulp. The enamel is extremely hard and protects the crown (the exposed portion of tooth above the gingiva) from injury and infection. The dentin layer comprises the largest portion of the tooth and, unlike the enamel, can regenerate. The pulp contains both the blood vessels and nerves from the crown through the root. The roots connect the tooth to the mandibular or maxillary neurovasculature. The root is embedded in the socket and attached via the periodontal ligament (**Fig. 1**). Upper teeth are attached to the alveolar bone of the maxilla, whereas lower teeth are connected to the mandibular alveolar bone.

The adult mouth is composed of 32 teeth, numbered from patient's right to left on the top and then from left to right on the bottom. Wisdom teeth may or may not have erupted in adults. Primary tooth eruption begins in most children around age 6 months (typically with the lower central incisors) and continues to the last molars by age 3 years. The 20 primary teeth are labeled with letters A through T (**Fig. 2**).

EXAMINATION

A thorough examination is important in patients presenting with facial pain or injury. Concomitant intracranial and maxillofacial injuries are present in up to 11% of patients presenting to the ED with dental trauma.[4] Sources of referred pain, such as temporal mandibular joint inflammation, otitis media, sinusitis, migraine headaches, and/or trigeminal neuralgia, can also cause dental pain and can usually be diagnosed with a thorough history and physical.[5] Airway patency is rarely an issue in dental emergencies; however, oropharyngeal bleeding, severe submandibular swelling, or aspirated dental fragments can impede the airway. Evaluation should include patient's phonation, swallowing, ability to clear secretions or blood, presence of stridor, and/or subjective foreign body sensation in throat or airway.

Intraoral examination includes inspection of teeth for fractures, as well as palpation for instability or tenderness. All intraoral tissues should also be inspected and palpated, including gingiva, buccal mucosa, tongue, frenulum, tonsils, and uvula. Note should be made of lacerations; abrasions; ecchymoses; foreign bodies, including tooth fragments; and any edema, masses, or signs of infection.

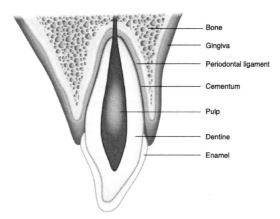

Fig. 1. Tooth anatomy. (*From* Piccininni P, Clough A, Padilla R, et al. Dental and orofacial injuries. Clin Sports Med 2017;36:369–405; with permission.)

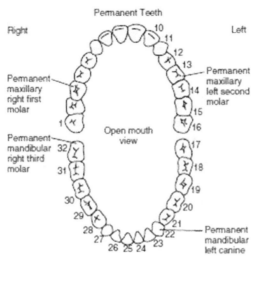

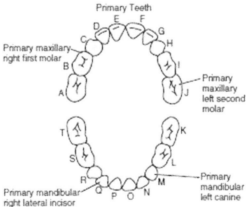

Fig. 2. Primary and permanent tooth numbering. (*From* Benko K. Dental procedures. In: Roberts JR, Custalow CB, Thomsen TW, et al, editors. Roberts and Hedges' clinical procedures in emergency medicine. Philadelphia: Elsevier; 2014; with permission.)

ATRAUMATIC DENTAL PAIN

Pain with tooth eruption, both primary and permanent, is common. Symptoms of teething, or primary tooth eruption, are generally mild to moderate and include localized discomfort, drooling, and occasionally fussiness. Conservative measures can be effective, such as acetaminophen, ibuprofen, and/or ice water or cool compresses to the area. Due to potential systemic toxicity from misuse, topical lidocaine preparations are no longer recommended in children. Fever is often attributed to teething but there is no proven relationship between tooth eruption and fever.[6] High fever, localized swelling, and/or drainage should raise concern about secondary infection. Pain with permanent tooth eruption is also common and occasionally complicated by pericoronitis, or infection of the gingiva, near the emerging tooth surface.

Dental pain can also be related to tooth extractions. Immediately after the extraction, patients experience moderate and sometimes severe localized pain. This is best treated with ice, nonsteroidal antiinflammatories (NSAIDS), acetaminophen, and perhaps a short course of oral opioids. Occasionally trismus can develop in the first day related to postprocedural edema and temporary muscle spasm.[7] If trismus is severe or worsening, infection or hematoma should be considered. Pain should be significantly improved within 48 hours unless alveolar osteitis is developing.

Several days after an extraction, when the clot is dislodged, an acute increase in pain can occur from dry socket, or postextraction alveolar osteitis. Despite its name, this is usually not infectious in cause but rather an inflammatory response of the newly exposed alveolar bone. It occurs in 3% to 4% of patients after tooth extractions, and smokers are at higher risk.[8] The symptoms respond well to NSAIDS, dental blocks, and gentle irrigation of the socket. Prompt referral to the practitioner who performed the extraction is warranted.

ORAL AND DENTAL TRAUMA

Dental trauma is extremely common, with approximately one-third of all people suffering a dental injury during their lifetime.[9,10] Maxillary incisors are the most commonly injured, with the central maxillary incisors at highest risk in children with significant overbites.[11-13] Male patients are more commonly injured than female patients, with falls and motor vehicle collisions being the most common mechanisms.[14]

Injuries include dental concussions, fractures of crown and/or root, luxation or loosening, and complete avulsions. Treatment depends mainly on the extent of the injury and whether the involved teeth are primary or permanent. The goal of the emergency provider is to identify all injuries, initiate treatment to preserve the function of the tooth, and prevent infection to the extent possible. For all injuries, prompt follow-up with a dentist should be arranged.

Dental Fractures

Fractures of the crown (the part visible above the gum line) are classified based on the depth of the fracture and by the Ellis system (**Fig. 3**). Ellis I fractures involve only the enamel. They are painless and do not bleed. These fractures require no emergent treatment other than routine referral to a dentist for cosmetic repair. Ellis II fractures involve the dentin and account for approximately 70% or all fractures.[7] These tend to be painful, as well as sensitive to extremes of temperature, and may bleed slightly. Ellis III fractures involve the pulp and pose the highest risk of pulp necrosis and/or infection, which threatens the integrity of the tooth. After bleeding is controlled by the application of pressure with sterile gauze, Ellis II and III fractures should be covered by temporary dental cement (calcium hydroxide preparation is commercially available and often part of prepared dental kits). Bleeding can also be controlled with application of tranexamic acid on a gauze pad if simple pressure does not suffice. A soft diet should be advised, with no biting on the side of the injured tooth. Prompt referral to a dentist is indicated. Prophylactic antibiotics are generally not needed.

Fractures of the root of the tooth and the alveolar socket can be harder to diagnose in the ED. It is often not possible to differentiate a simply concussed tooth from a root fracture because they both may be somewhat tender and minimally loose on examination. Patients should be referred to their dentist so that radiographs can be performed. Root fractures closer to the crown of the tooth carry a worse prognosis for long-term viability of the tooth.[11]

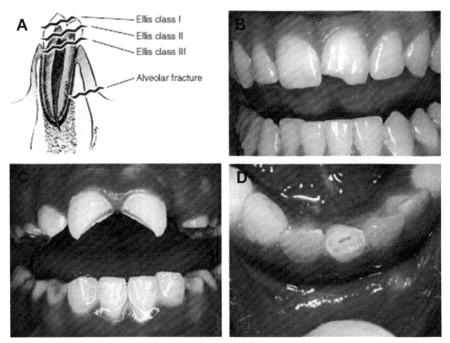

Fig. 3. Ellis fractures. (*From* Benko K. Dental procedures. In: Roberts JR, Custalow CB, Thomsen TW, et al, editors. Roberts and Hedges' clinical procedures in emergency medicine. Philadelphia: Elsevier; 2014; with permission.)

Tooth Displacement or Luxation

Teeth can be luxated (loosened) with or without fractures. The goal of treatment of these injuries is to stabilize the teeth and preserve their blood supply. Concussion is the most minor type of injury, defined by tenderness to palpation secondary to subclinical loosening but without disruption of the periodontal ligament. Luxation is palpable loosening that can be intrusive, extrusive, lateral, or a combination. The treatment of luxation varies based on whether the tooth is primary or permanent, and in what direction the tooth is displaced. In primary teeth, the main concern is preserving the integrity of the alveolar bone for the future eruption of permanent teeth. For this reason, loosened primary teeth should not be forcibly pushed back into the socket. If there is no or little resistance, the tooth can be gently repositioned and splinted to adjacent teeth. Parents should be counseled that the tooth may not reimplant successfully but that long-term cosmesis and growth of the permanent tooth should be unaffected.

Permanent teeth that have been loosened should generally be gently reduced back into anatomic position. Extruded teeth (partially pulled out of the socket) should be promptly reduced to preserve neurovascular integrity (**Fig. 4**). Immature permanent teeth with developing, open apices have the greatest chance of survival after extrusive luxation, whereas fully formed teeth are at greater risk of pulp necrosis.[15] After reduction, the tooth is assumed to still be unstable and should be splinted with wax or dental cement to the 2 adjacent teeth. If there is significant resistance to reducing an extruded tooth, there may be a hematoma or clot in the socket. The physician can pad the tooth with gauze and instruct the patient to bite down very gently.[16] Too

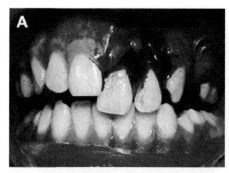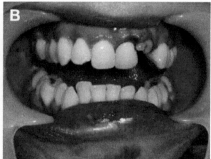

Fig. 4. Tooth luxation: (A) extrusive luxation, (B) intrusive luxation. (*Adapted from* Piccininni P, Clough A, Padilla R, et al. Dental and orofacial injuries. Clin Sports Med 2017;36:369–405; with permission.)

much pressure risks causing a fracture at the root or the socket. A dentist or oral surgeon should be involved if reduction is unsuccessful after these maneuvers.

Intrusive luxation occurs when the tooth is forcibly pushed deeper into the socket. This is fairly uncommon, comprising only 2% of all dental injuries but almost 70% of intrusive luxation injuries involve the central maxillary incisors[17] (see **Fig. 4**). Significant damage can be done to the tooth itself, particularly the root, as well as the alveolar bone and periodontal ligament, making long-term tooth viability challenging. Though no ED management is indicated other than appropriate pain control, patients need prompt dental follow-up. The dentist will manage these with either close monitoring for reeruption (more likely in primary teeth), surgical repositioning with or without root canal, or extraction of the tooth.

Complete avulsion of a tooth is a common injury. The avulsed tooth should be gently rinsed (not scrubbed) in saline then stored in saline, milk, or saliva and transported with the patient. If the tooth cannot be found, it may be embedded in oral lacerations, aspirated, swallowed, or lost at the scene. Chest radiograph may be performed to assess for aspiration of the tooth. This can occur without respiratory compromise and, if left undetected, can lead to pulmonary infection.

Avulsed primary teeth should never be replaced. Not only would they be physically difficult to replace but, more importantly, attempts at replacement can damage the alveolar socket and developing permanent tooth. Routine dental follow-up is recommended to ensure proper healing of the socket. Permanent teeth should be replaced as quickly as possible. Exceptions to this recommendation include a tooth with severe dental caries, an uncooperative patient, immunosuppression, or patients with mechanical heart valves.[18] The tooth should be rinsed with saline to remove clot but, to avoid damage to the periodontal ligament, it should not be scrubbed. The tooth should be gently reduced into anatomic position and splinted to the 2 adjacent teeth with dental cement or wax. Close follow-up should be arranged with the dentist for definitive bridging and repair.

Dental Bleeding

Most oropharyngeal bleeding is self-limited and due to either trauma or dental procedures. As with most soft tissue bleeding, steady direct pressure for 10 to 15 minutes is the first-line therapy. Next, local injection of lidocaine with epinephrine can help vasoconstrict the area, then direct pressure is again applied. Another therapy that shows promise is topical tranexamic acid.[19] The same formulation that is used intravenously

(500 mg in 10 mL of saline), is applied to gauze or cotton. This is then held with pressure on the bleeding site or the patient can gently bite down on the gauze.

If these measures fail, the extraction site may need to be sutured in a figure 8 fashion to achieve hemostasis. Reversal of any anticoagulation, inherent coagulopathy, and/or an antiplatelet agent should be considered if there is continued bleeding. Finally, if the patient continues to bleed significantly, there may have been injury to an artery, vein, or arteriovenous malformation. Involvement of the oral surgeon is appropriate at this point, as well as interventional radiology to consider either surgical management or embolization.[8]

Dental Infections

Dental infections range from simple caries to more severe abscesses and necrotizing gingivitis. Caries is the breakdown of tooth enamel caused by plaque and oral flora. It is treated with pain management and requires a referral to a dentist for excavation and filling.[8] Antibiotics are generally not indicated.

Pulpitis is inflammation of the pulp cavity of a tooth where the neurovascular structures are located.[8] Pulpitis can be caused by caries, trauma, recent dental procedures, defective fillings, and chemical toxins.[20] Pulpitis presents as dental pain exacerbated by extremes of temperature.[20] Initially, pulpitis can be reversible but with time can become irreversible. Treatment involves filling of the dental cavity and root canal. Antibiotics generally do not play a role.[21]

Pulpitis, if severe and untreated, can erode into the dentoalveolar ridge and cause a periapical abscess (**Fig. 5**). This requires drainage and either dental extraction or root canal and repair of dental caries. Antibiotics alone will not suffice but should be started until the patient can see a dentist.

A periodontal abscess develops from spread of local infection from the supportive dental structures, such as the gums and dental ligament. Gingivitis is the initial reversible stage of gum inflammation characterized by erythema, swelling, and edema from plaque buildup[20] (**Fig. 6**). As gingivitis progresses, periodontitis can develop. This is irreversible inflammation and destruction of the supporting structures. Areas of bone loss can become infected and progress to a periodontal abscess. In contrast to periapical abscess, teeth surrounded by a periodontal abscess may be entirely healthy without underlying pulpitis or carious change.

Some gingival abscesses are amenable to incision and drainage in the ED or needle aspiration as a temporizing measure. Imaging is generally not needed. Computed tomography may be useful to assess for complications such as submandibular abscess, cavernous sinus thrombosis, dental fistula, maxillary sinusitis, or preseptal or postseptal cellulitis.[22]

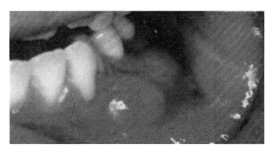

Fig. 5. Periapical abscess. (*From* Hodgdon A. Dental and related infections. Emerg Med Clin 2013;31(2):465–80; with permission.)

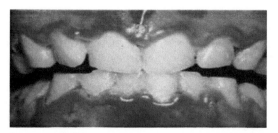

Fig. 6. Gingivitis. (*From* Hodgdon A. Dental and related infections. Emerg Med Clin 2013;31(2):465–80; with permission.)

Pericoronitis is inflammation and infection of the gingiva around teeth as they erupt due to impaction and irritation from food particles. Pain and infection are particularly common with wisdom teeth.[23] Often, a wisdom tooth erupts without an opposing tooth, making chewing difficult and the tooth more prone to food becoming caught with subsequent dental caries and/or pericoronitis. Like other forms of gingivitis, this localized inflammation can vary from mild to superinfection with significant spread. The prevalence of pericoronitis is 80% in patients aged 20 to 29 years.[24] Initial treatment focuses on meticulous oral hygiene, whereas definitive management for persistent symptoms includes molar extraction. Antibiotics are reserved for cases in which surgical intervention is delayed or in which systemic symptoms are present.[24]

A final notable dental infection is acute necrotizing ulcerative gingivitis (ANUG), also known as Vincent disease and trench mouth.[25] ANUG is seen primarily in immunosuppressed patients or in developing countries, and is due to malnutrition and poor oral hygiene.[25] When ANUG is suspected in an otherwise healthy patient, human immunodeficiency virus (HIV) infection should be considered. ANUG has a prevalence of 4.3% to 16% in HIV-infected patients.[26] The infection is polymicrobial in nature, including *Bacteroides*, fusiform (*Bacillus*), and spirochetes.[26,27] The diagnosis of ANUG is based on clinical findings, most commonly necrosis and ulceration of the interdental papilla, gingival bleeding, pain (often rapid in onset), and pseudomembrane formation[27] (**Fig. 7**). Treatment includes oral care and debridement of the necrotic tissue. Though antibiotics are indicated for systemic symptoms, the mainstay of therapy is improved oral hygiene.

Procedures

Before performing any dental procedure, the clinician must assess the risk of airway compromise and be prepared for any complication. Airway obstruction and/or

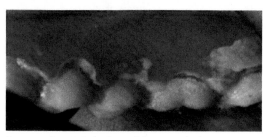

Fig. 7. Pseudomembranes of ANUG. (*Adapted from* Hodgdon A. Dental and related infections. Emerg Med Clin 2013;31(2):465–80; with permission.)

aspiration can result from redundant anatomy, loose teeth, bleeding, loose dental instruments, and purulent material.

Appropriate anesthesia is key for patient comfort, as well as to allow adequate time for the operator to perform the procedure successfully.[28] Anesthetics may be topical or injected. Topical medications are typically used for noninvasive or minimally invasive procedures. Topical medications typically require several minutes of contact time with the oral mucosa to achieve anesthetic effect. Topical medications are available in gel, liquid, aerosol, and ointment forms. Most contain benzocaine 20% and exhibit no systemic absorption.[28]

Lidocaine is the prototypical amide anesthetic. When epinephrine is added to the lidocaine the anesthetic effects are longer and higher doses are tolerated before any toxicity.[28] Mepivacaine and prilocaine are intermediate-duration amide anesthetics, lasting approximately 2 to 3 hours, similar to lidocaine with epinephrine. Bupivacaine is a long-acting amide anesthetic with a duration of action of 6 to 8 hours. This makes it ideal for ED dental blocks to provide prolonged analgesia for patients with dental pain.

A very useful and common procedure is to anesthetize an individual tooth by supraperiosteal injection. The mucobuccal fold should be exposed by grasping the lip or cheek and pulling up and out for mandibular teeth, or down and out for maxillary teeth. The fold is entered with a 25-gauge needle, aspirated, and 1 to 2 mL of local anesthetic is delivered to the bone of the respective tooth being anesthetized (**Fig. 8**). It may take several minutes for the anesthetic to penetrate the bone and reach the nerve.

Another useful nerve block is the inferior alveolar nerve block, which anesthetizes the ipsilateral mandibular teeth to the midline, the buccal mucosa anterior to the first molar, and the skin and mucosa of the lower lip. This nerve block can be challenging to perform properly. The goal is to place the anesthetic between the internal oblique ridge of the mandible (laterally) and the pterygomandibular raphe (medially).[29]

The external oblique ridge can be palpated by placing the nondominant thumb into the patient's mouth. With the same hand, the index finger is placed external to the mouth behind the ramus of the mandible and the cheek is retracted laterally. This serves 2 purposes: it makes the tissue taut and exposes the pterygomandibular triangle for injection, and it removes the operator's fingers from the teeth and needle tip.[30] With the dominant hand, grasp the syringe and deliver the 25-gauge needle tip to the landmark from the contralateral premolars, with the needle held parallel to the occlusal plane of the teeth (**Fig. 9**). The needle should be inserted until bone is felt, approximately 20 to 25 mm in depth, and approximately 1 cm above the occlusal surface of the molars. Once bone is felt, the needle should be withdrawn 1 to 2 mm and aspirated for blood. If no blood is noted, 1 to 2 mL of anesthetic should be deposited into the tissue.[30]

To anesthetize the maxillary teeth, several nerve blocks may be performed. The molars can be anesthetized by the posterior superior alveolar nerve (PSAN) and the middle superior alveolar nerve (MSAN) blocks. The PSAN block may not completely anesthetize the ipsilateral first molar, which is why the MSAN block may be useful.[30] To perform the PSAN block, have the patient close his or her mouth halfway and deviate the jaw laterally toward the side of the injection. Grasp the cheek and pull it laterally. The 25-gauge needle should puncture the maxillary mucosa just distal to the second molar (**Fig. 10**). The needle should be directed superiorly and posteriorly to a depth of 2 to 2.5 cm then 2 to 3 mL of anesthetic should be delivered.[30]

The MSAN block is used to assure complete anesthesia of the maxillary first molar. The anterior superior alveolar nerve (ASAN) block is used to anesthetize the canine and the incisors on the ipsilateral side. The blocks are done in an identical manner

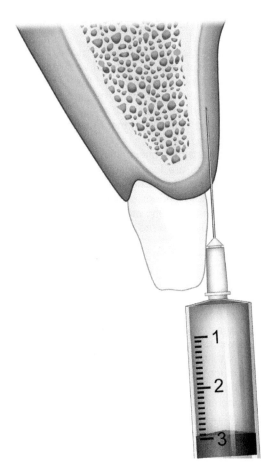

Fig. 8. Supraperiosteal injection technique. (*Adapted from* Benko K. Dental procedures. In: Roberts JR, Custalow CB, Thomsen TW, et al, editors. Roberts and Hedges' clinical procedures in emergency medicine. Philadelphia: Elsevier; 2014; with permission.)

but with different maxillary teeth as landmarks. To perform the MSAN block, the needle puncture is at the second premolar mucobuccal fold, at a 45-degree angle to the bone. The ASAN block is performed in the same manner but at the canine (see **Fig. 10**). In each procedure, 2 mL of anesthetic is deposited.[30]

Special Considerations

In addition to attending to immediate oropharyngeal injuries and infections, there are certain at-risk populations and special considerations the emergency provider should also take into account. First, nonaccidental trauma and neglect are concerns in the pediatric and geriatric populations, as well as in the cognitively impaired. Typical injuries in children include falls forward with injuries to anterior incisors, chin, and lips. Injuries to the angle of the mandible or the molars should raise concern for abuse if the mechanism is incongruent with the injury.

Dental injuries can also provide an opportunity for the emergency provider to counsel parents regarding injury prevention, including gating staircases and padding

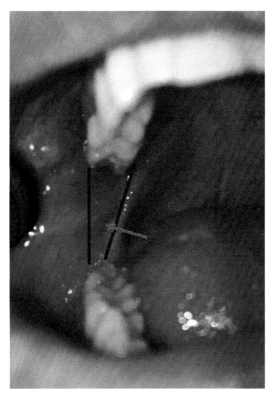

Fig. 9. Pterygomandibular triangle with needle insertion point (*blue arrow*) for inferior alveolar nerve block.

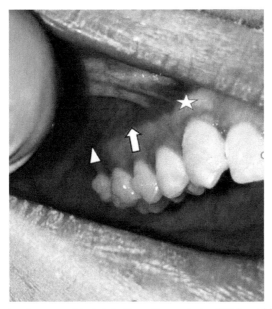

Fig. 10. Superior alveolar nerve block injection sites: anterior (*star*), middle (*arrow*), posterior (*arrowhead*).

the corners of furniture for toddlers, and mouthguard use in older children. Sports account for up to 39% of all dental injuries in children.[31] Use of a mouthguard decreases the risk of dental injury by 5% to 20%.[32] The mouthguard is a rubber or plastic device that covers the upper, and occasionally the lower, teeth and serves to dissipate energy from a blow to the teeth or lips to avoid lip laceration and tooth injuries.[33]

SUMMARY

Dental complaints, typically infections, injuries, and pain, are common reasons for patients to seek care in the ED. In trauma, the goal is to preserve the viability of the tooth, maximize cosmesis, and do no damage to the underlying alveolar bone and developing permanent tooth in young children. With dental infections, many times the role of the ED is to temporize until definitive dental extraction can be performed or, in severe cases of spreading oropharyngeal infection, assessing the need for intravenous antibiotics and/or surgical drainage. For most issues, pain is a major concern. As discussed, NSAIDS and dental blocks can be extremely effective. The principles outlined in this article will help guide the emergency provider in the proper diagnosis and management of these issues.

REFERENCES

1. Lewis C, Lynch H, Johnston B. Dental complaints in emergency departments: a national perspective. Ann Emerg Med 2003;42:93–9.
2. Kman NE. Dental emergencies. In: Sherman SC, et al, editors. Clinical emergency medicine. New York: McGraw-Hill; 2014 [Chapter: 78].
3. Richardson LD, Hwang U. Access to care: a review of the emergency medicine literature. Acad Emerg Med 2001;8:1030–6.
4. Nalliah RP, Allareddy V, Elangovan S, et al. Hospital based emergency department visits attributed to dental caries in the United States in 2006. J Evid Based Dent Pract 2010;10:212–22.
5. Okeson JP, Falace DA. Nonodontogenic toothache. Dent Clin North Am 1997;41: 367–83.
6. Kiran K, Swati T, Kamala BK, et al. Prevalence of systemic and local disturbances in infants during primary teeth eruption: a clinical study. Eur J Paediatr Dent 2011; 12:249–52.
7. Beaudreau RW. Oral and dental emergencies. In: Tintinalli JE, et al, editors. Tintinalli's emergency medicine: a comprehensive study guide. 8th edition. New York: McGraw Hill; 2015 [Chapter: 245].
8. Deangelis AF. Review article: maxillofacial emergencies: oral pain and odontogenic infections. Emerg Med Australas 2014;26:336–42.
9. Moule A, Cohenca N. Emergency assessment and treatment planning for traumatic dental injuries. Aust Dent J 2016;61(1 suppl):21–38.
10. Nalliah RP, Rampa S, Lee MK, et al. Epidemiology and outcomes of hospital-based emergency visits with tooth fractures. Pediatr Dent 2015;37:348–54.
11. Piccininni P, Clough A, Padilla R, et al. Dental and orofacial injuries. Clin Sports Med 2017;36:369–405.
12. Atabek D, Alaçam A, Aydintuğ I, et al. A retrospective study of traumatic dental injuries. Dent Traumatol 2014;30:154–61.
13. Francisco SS, Filho FJ, Pinheiro ET, et al. Prevalence of traumatic dental injuries and associated factors among Brazilian schoolchildren. Oral Health Prev Dent 2013;11:31–8.

14. Bastone EB, Freer TJ, McNamara JR. Epidemiology of dental trauma: a review of the literature. Aust Dent J 2000;45:2–9.
15. Sigurdsson A, Bourguignon C. Traumatic injuries to athletes. Gen Dent 2015;63: 24–9.
16. Ross DJ. Subluxed and avulsed tooth management. In: Reichman EF, editor. Emergency medicine procedures. 2nd edition. New York: McGraw-Hill; 2013 [Chapter 181].
17. Omar S, Freccia WF, Retamozo B, et al. Traumatically intruded permanent teeth: three case reports and a review of current recommendations. J Calif Dent Assoc 2017;45:245–53.
18. International Association of Dental Traumatology. Dental trauma guidelines, revised 2012. Available at: https://www.iadt-dentaltrauma.org/1-9%20%20iadt% 20guidelines%20combined%20-%20lr%20-%2011-5-2013.pdf. Accessed August 13, 2018.
19. Flynn TR. Principles of management of odontogenic infections. In: Miloro M, et al, editors. Peterson's principles of oral and maxillofacial surgery. 2nd edition. London: BC Decker; 2004 [Chapter: 15].
20. Hodgdon A. Dental and related infections. Emerg Med Clin North Am 2013;31: 465–80.
21. Agnihotry A, Fedorowicz Z, van Zuuren EJ, et al. Antibiotic use for irreversible pulpitis. Cochrane Database Syst Rev 2016;(2):CD004969.
22. Shuaib W, Hashmi M, Vijayasarathi A, et al. The use of facial CT for the evaluation of a suspected simple dentoalveolar abscess in the emergency department. Clin Med Res 2015;13:112–6.
23. Douglass AB, Douglass JM. Common dental emergencies. Am Fam Physician 2003;67:511–6.
24. Renton T, Wilson NH. Problems with erupting wisdom teeth: signs, symptoms, and management. Br J Gen Pract 2016;66:e606–8.
25. Folayan MO. The epidemiology, etiology, and pathophysiology of acute necrotizing ulcerative gingivitis associated with malnutrition. J Contemp Dent Pract 2004;5:28–41.
26. Shangase L, Feller L, Blignaut E. Necrotising ulcerative gingivitis/periodontitis as indicators of HIV-infection. SADJ 2004;59:105–8.
27. Herrera D, Retamal-Valdes B, Alonso B, et al. Acute periodontal lesions (periodontal abscesses and necrotizing periodontal diseases) and endo-periodontal lesions. J Clin Periodontol 2018;45:S78–94.
28. Ogle OE, Mahjoubi G. Local anesthesia: agents, techniques, and complications. Dent Clin North Am 2012;56:133–48.
29. Virdee SS, Seymour D, Bhakta S. Effective anaesthesia of the acutely inflamed pulp: part 1. The acutely inflamed pulp. Br Dent J 2015;219:385–90.
30. Benko K. Dental procedures. In: Roberts JR, Custalow CB, Thomsen TW, et al, editors. Roberts and Hedges' clinical procedures in emergency medicine. Philadelphia: Elsevier; 2014.
31. Newsome PR, Tran DC, Cooke MS. The role of the mouthguard in the prevention of sports-related dental injuries: a review. Int J Paediatr Dent 2001;11:396–404.
32. Knapik JJ, Marshall SW, Lee RB, et al. Mouthguards in sports activities: history, physical properties and injury prevention effectiveness. Sports Med 2007;37: 117–44.
33. Parker K, Marlow B, Patel N, et al. A review of mouthguards: effectiveness, types, characteristics and indications for use. Br Dent J 2017;222:629–33.

Infections of the Neck

Renjie Michael Li, MD[a], Michael Kiemeney, MD[b],*

KEYWORDS

- Peritonsillar abscess • Pharyngitis • Retropharyngeal abscess • Lemierre syndrome
- Descending necrotizing mediastinitis • Ludwig angina • Epiglottitis
- Deep space neck infections

KEY POINTS

- Retropharyngeal abscess may present, similarly to meningitis, with fever and neck stiffness. A high index of suspicion, as well as signs of airway or pharyngeal involvement, should lead to computed tomography imaging and the correct diagnosis.
- Septic patients with oropharyngeal involvement and concomitant distant infections, such as pulmonary abscess or septic arthritis, should increase concern for Lemierre syndrome.
- Pharyngitis with a positive rapid *Streptococcus* antigen detection test and 2 or more Centor criteria should be treated. Neither test nor treat patients with 0 or 1 Centor criteria.
- The epidemiology of epiglottitis has shifted to a rare presentation in young children but should still be considered in unvaccinated children and young adults.

INTRODUCTION

The neck is a complex, enclosed structure best assessed by palpation. Anterior landmarks include the cricoid cartilage in adults and the hyoid bone in children. Laterally, the neck is loosely divided into the anterior and posterior triangles, with the sternocleidomastoid separating them. Internally, the neck is bounded by the hollow spaces that are also themselves divisible into the nasopharynx, the oral cavity, the oropharynx, and the larynx. The nasopharynx runs from the base of the skull to the soft palate. The oral cavity extends from the lips to the anterior two-thirds of the tongue. The oropharynx extends from the posterior one-third of the tongue to the vallecula. The larynx comprises 3 compartments: the supraglottis, including the epiglottis and false vocal cords; the glottis, inclusive of the true vocal cords and arytenoids; and the subglottis, which extends to the margin of the cricoid cartilage. Between these external and internal landmarks is a structure rich in nerves and vasculature and intricately compartmentalized

Dr R.M. Li and Dr M. Kiemeney have no financial interests to disclose.
[a] Department of Emergency Medicine, Loma Linda University Medical Center, 11234 Anderson Street MC A-108, Loma Linda, CA 92354, USA; [b] Department of Emergency Medicine, Loma Linda University School of Medicine, 11234 Anderson Street MC A-108, Loma Linda, CA 92354, USA
* Corresponding author.
E-mail address: mkiemeney@llu.edu

Emerg Med Clin N Am 37 (2019) 95–107
https://doi.org/10.1016/j.emc.2018.09.003
0733-8627/19/© 2018 Elsevier Inc. All rights reserved.
emed.theclinics.com

by fascial layers. The surgical otolaryngology literature outlines the deep neck spaces into 13 separate compartments, illustrating the complexity of this anatomy.[1] However, what is apparent is that infections that begin in 1 area of the neck can travel rapidly within their respective fascial planes. Because of limited space to allow for swelling, deep neck infections can swiftly progress. This has serious implications for delays in treatment, including airway compromise; necrosis of surrounding structures; and contiguous spread to other compartments, such as the mediastinum.

PHARYNGITIS (TONSILLITIS)

Pharyngitis and tonsillitis are common presenting complaints in the emergency department (ED) accounting for more than 14 million visits annually to clinics, urgent care settings, and EDs.[2] The pathophysiology of acute pharyngitis or tonsillitis is relatively straightforward. It is thought to be either the localized inflammation of direct viral or bacterial invasion into the superficial oropharyngeal mucosa or the secondary inflammation caused by nasal secretions running down the nasopharynx. Current practice patterns contribute to an economic burden in the United States worth an estimated 1.2 billion dollars and close to half of that can be reduced by adherence to clinical guidelines, reducing antibiotic prescriptions, resistance, and return visits.[3]

Viral pharyngitis (and tonsillitis) is more common than bacterial pharyngitis and, although the viral course is generally self-limited, bacterial pharyngitis caused by Group A streptococcus (GAS) can cause more serious, nonsuppurative complications, such as rheumatic fever, with or without carditis and poststreptococcal glomerulonephritis. GAS is largely a disease of children 5 to 15 years old, living in temperate climates, in the months between the start of winter and spring. This population composes approximately 20% to 30% of all cases of infectious pharyngitis in children and 5% to 15% of cases in adults. Treatment of viral pharyngitis is supportive with the goal of symptom relief. However, antibiotics are reportedly prescribed in up to 70% of patients presenting to primary care practices with symptoms consistent with pharyngitis.[4] The pitfall in clinical practice is that symptoms alone cannot adequately differentiate viral versus bacterial pharyngitis and laboratory testing, such as the rapid Streptococcus antigen test, is only 70% to 90% sensitive when compared with pharyngeal culture, which is the current gold standard.[5] Additionally, there is also a large proportion of the population who are chronic GAS carriers. This is estimated to be 5% to 25% of the population.[6]

Many clinical decision tools have been introduced to guide antibiotic use but the most widely used was published in 1981 by Robert Centor.[7] The Centor criteria are simple, with 4 aspects of clinical presentation making Streptococcus pharyngitis more likely. These are: history of fever; lack of cough; presence of tonsillar exudates; and tender, anterior cervical adenopathy. However, the interpretation of the Centor criteria has changed through the years. The current Infectious Diseases Society of America (IDSA) guideline recommends neither testing nor treatment of those patients who present with 1 or 0 criteria, and then only treatment of rapid Streptococcus antigen detection test (RADT)-positive individuals with 2 or more Centor criteria. For older children and adolescents, negative RADT testing should be backed up by confirmatory throat culture. GAS testing is not recommended for children younger than 3 years old due to an extremely low incidence of rheumatic fever in that age group. Routine culture is also not recommended for RADT-negative adults because the incidence of GAS pharyngitis in adults is 10% and the risk of rheumatic fever is exceedingly low for adults. The IDSA advises no testing for pharyngitis that is clearly viral with associated symptoms such as coryza, conjunctivitis, stomatitis, cough, rash, or diarrhea.[3,4,8] Treatment of streptococcus pharyngitis is penicillin or amoxicillin because of their narrow-spectrum coverage and cost-effectiveness. Alternative antibiotics include first-generation cephalosporins, clindamycin, or macrolides.[4] Treatment of viral pharyngitis is generally supportive. Steroids are not recommended by the IDSA. However, there have been multiple randomized controlled trials (RCTs) demonstrating that steroids may shorten the course and severity of the illness. These RCTs show significant pain reduction in acute pharyngitis with steroid administration, although the route of administration seems to be inconsequential (oral vs parenteral).[9–11]

EPIGLOTTITIS (SUPRAGLOTTITIS)

Epiglottitis is a cellulitis of the epiglottis, as well as of the surrounding tissue that lie between it and the false vocal cords (**Fig. 1**). It is still a feared presentation in emergency medicine because the supraglottic tissue can become severely edematous, extending posteriorly and inferiorly, compressing the vocal cords. Acute obstruction can also happen with mucous plugging or laryngospasm of the already narrowed airway. After the introduction of the conjugated *Haemophilus influenzae* type B (Hib) vaccine in 1987, supraglottitis in children nearly vanished, with an incidence of 3.47 per 100,000 in 1980 to 0.63 per 100,000 in 1990. However, the incidence in adults remained relatively stable, thus pushing the median age of presentation toward older children and young adults.[12] The causative organism has also shifted to a predominance of *Streptococcus*, *Staphylococcus*, and nontypeable *Haemophilus* spp.[13]

The diagnosis of epiglottitis requires a high degree of clinical suspicion. Especially in the early stages, it can present like pharyngitis, tonsillitis, or croup, particularly in the pediatric population. The classic presentation, however, is a toxic-appearing patient with dysphagia, stridor, or drooling. Adults usually present less acutely due to larger airways that allow for more swelling. Symptoms in adults may begin as more tolerable complaints, such as sore throat, odynophagia, and voice changes. The general principle when examining a patient with suspected epiglottitis, especially the pediatric patient, is to avoid interventions that can provoke anxiety in the patient, such as unnecessary laboratory draws, frequent repositioning, intravenous (IV) access, or direct examination with a tongue depressor. If the clinical examination is nondiagnostic, a few imaging modalities can be considered. A computed tomography (CT) scan is not likely to be well-tolerated because it requires the patient to lie flat. A portable lateral soft tissue neck plain film can be used when available. The pathognomonic

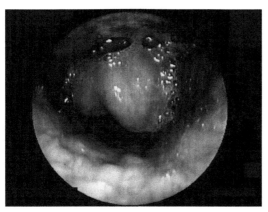

Fig. 1. Epiglottitis on endoscopy. (*From* Wikimedia Commons; 2013. Available at: https://en.wikipedia.org/wiki/File:Epiglottitis_endoscopy.jpg. Accessed June 2, 2018.)

thumb-print sign can be a specific diagnostic finding; however, the sensitivity of plain films is lacking (76%) and should not override clinical judgment.[14] Bedside ultrasound may be a quick, efficient, and reliable diagnostic modality in the ED; however, there is still a lack of large trials demonstrating ultrasound sensitivity and specificity in the diagnosis of epiglottitis. One small study demonstrated the accuracy of ultrasound measurements in laryngoscope-confirmed epiglottitis, although other studies have shown that ultrasound can reliably measure the width of the epiglottis.[15,16] When epiglottitis is suspected, anesthesiology or otolaryngology should be consulted early in the patient's clinical course. Ideally, the airway will be secured in the operating room with advanced modalities such as flexible fiberoptic scope and surgical airway intervention on standby.

Antibiotics should be initiated with a third-generation cephalosporin, with the addition of vancomycin in methicillin-resistant *Staphylococcus aureus* (MRSA)-suspected cases. In patients allergic to penicillin, levofloxacin can be used.[17] Although dexamethasone is frequently given to decrease airway inflammation and swelling, there is little evidence to support its use.[18]

PERITONSILLAR ABSCESS

A disease of the oropharynx, peritonsillar abscess (PTA) is the most common deep neck infection in adults.[19] Usually seen in young to middle-aged adults, PTA can be included in the spectrum of tonsillitis. Clinical presentation may include sore throat, hoarse voice, trismus, fever, malaise, and food intolerance. Physical examination often shows a deviated uvula with an area of fluctuance abutting an inflamed tonsil, which may be obscured depending on size (**Fig. 2**). PTA is a bread-and-butter ED complaint that is often treated with a relatively simple procedural drainage via surgical incision or needle aspiration. However, if not treated properly, it is susceptible to complications

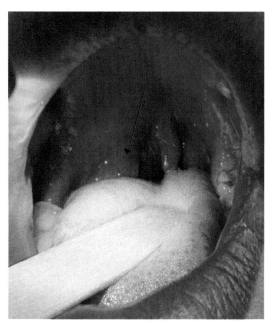

Fig. 2. Peritonsillar abscess (*arrow*). (*From* Wikimedia Commons. Available at: https://commons.wikimedia.org/wiki/File:PeritonsilarAbsess.jpg. Accessed June 2, 2018.)

such as airway obstruction, aspiration of abscess contents, necrosis into the carotid sheath, and further extension into the deep neck spaces.[20,21] The pathophysiology is not yet certain and is controversial but it is suspected to be a complication of bacterial tonsillar cellulitis. Proposed risk factors include tobacco, poor oral hygiene, and recent antibiotic use.[22] Aspirates from abscesses show a predominance of polymicrobial infections with a high incidence of GAS and anaerobes.[23] It is the common practice of many practitioners to treat with a course of antibiotics with anaerobic coverage after successful drainage of the abscess. However, a large RCT assessing the benefits of antibiotics is still lacking.[24] A single intravenous dose of dexamethasone has been shown to be effective in decreasing pain, as well as decreasing hospital stay and expediting tolerance of oral food or liquid.[25,26] Finally, the method of drainage remains an area of controversy in the literature. A Cochrane review performed in 2016 suggested that there is still no high-quality evidence for a superior outcome between needle aspiration and incision and drainage but conceded that smaller studies have demonstrated that incision and drainage may have marginally decreased recurrence rates and needle aspiration has some benefit in increasing patient comfort.[27]

LUDWIG ANGINA

Ludwig angina[28] was first described in 1836 by the German physician, Wilhelm Frederick von Ludwig as a gangrenous cellulitis involving the floor of the mouth and the neck. The term *angina* can be misleading because the chest pain that was initially described is not from cardiogenic causes but rather from the late complication of descending mediastinitis.[29] Ludwig angina is bilateral in nature, spread through contiguous tissue rather than lymphatics, and involves both the sublingual and submandibular spaces. It is generally odontogenic in origin (70%–90% of cases in various reports) and commonly arises from an infection of the second or third molars.[30] However, it can also be caused by oral trauma, oral mucosal breakdown, and foreign bodies such as piercings.[31] A retrospective analysis of reported cases found high rates of comorbidities, including diabetes mellitus, hypertension, and human immunodeficiency virus (HIV) infection. Other reported associated factors include dental infections and alcoholism, as well as patients who have undergone transplants or sustained trauma.[29] The classic presentation of Ludwig angina is a patient who complains of a rapidly swollen neck that may be tender to palpation. The neck is often described as brawny (ie, indurated to a tight, almost muscular, consistency). There is elevation of the floor of the mouth and protrusion of the tongue, indicating sublingual involvement. Other symptoms and examination findings may include fever, trismus, drooling, stridor, or frank airway obstruction.

The diagnosis of Ludwig angina is clinical. In the stable patient, CT scan and ultrasound can be helpful in confirming the diagnosis or assessing the degree of edema and risk of airway compromise. Treatment generally includes admission to an intensive care unit for airway monitoring and the immediate initiation of broad-spectrum antibiotics with coverage for oral flora. Early consultation by otolaryngology or anesthesia should be initiated when there is clinical suspicion of Ludwig angina because awake fiberoptic laryngoscopy or tracheostomy may be needed in the operating room. There is also very limited evidence for steroid and nebulized epinephrine use to delay surgical intervention; however, this has not been revisited with larger or newer studies.[31,32]

RETROPHARYNGEAL ABSCESS

The retropharyngeal space extends from the skull base to the tracheal bifurcation and lies anterior to the prevertebral fascia. Two paramedian chains of lymph nodes drain the nasopharynx, adenoids, and posterior nasal sinuses. Retropharyngeal abscesses

(RPAs) in pediatric patients typically arise from suppurative paramedian lymph nodes, with an incidence of 4.6 cases per 100,000 children. RPA in adults more commonly develop by direct extension from adjacent structures or direct inoculation due to trauma.[33]

RPA is a challenging diagnosis and most cases do not present with typical symptoms. Hoffman and colleagues[34] reported presenting symptoms in pediatric subjects as fever (100%), pain (100%), neck stiffness or torticollis (86%), neck swelling (68%), oropharyngeal bulging (67%), dysphagia (63%), trismus (11%), and dyspnea (2%). Other symptoms commonly encountered in pediatric patients are decreased oral intake, drooling, and odynophagia.[33]

The diagnostic gold standard is a CT scan with intravenous contrast.[35] A survey of pediatric ear, nose and throat (ENT) surgeons in 1999 showed that 72% preferred contrast-enhanced CT scan as their test of choice in the diagnostic evaluation of RPA.[36] Although considered to be the test of choice, contrast CT is not always definitive. False-positive and false-negative rates have been reported in the range of 10%.[33] Globally, CT scan abnormalities resulting in a diagnosis of RPA have a sensitivity of 43% to 89%, specificity of 0% to 63%, a positive predictive value (PPV) of 71% to 82%, and a negative predictive value (NPV) of 53% to 100%.[34] Ultrasound has been studied and in a case series was noted to be 100% specific and 53% sensitive, with a PPV of 96% and NPV of 16%.[37] Ultrasound may have equivalent sensitivity and greater specificity than CT scan in the diagnosis of pediatric RPA.

Treatment includes immediate ENT consultation for surgical drainage, IV hydration, and antibiotics. Recently, medical management of RPA has been gaining favor. A study using the KIDS' Inpatient Database compared a study cohort of 42.1% of subjects with RPA who underwent surgical treatment versus 57.9% treated nonsurgically. Dyspnea and/or stridor were found to have an odds ratio (OR) of 2.6 and streptococcal infection had an OR of 1.6 for surgical intervention. Fever (OR 0.6) and lymphadenopathy (OR 0.5) were associated with medical management.[38] Another case series of 178 subjects found two-thirds of subjects were managed medically and one-third had either immediate (<24 hours) or delayed (>24 hours) surgical intervention. The length of hospital stay for those patients who were medically managed (3 days) was nearly half that of those undergoing surgical treatment (5.5 days). This study showed the following factors are associated with the need for surgical intervention: age younger than 15 months, white blood cell count greater than 20.7, intensive care unit admission, CT findings of complete abscess, and abscess size greater than 2.2 cm.[39] Guidelines to define the patient population that would benefit from medical management have not been developed yet.

Medical management should focus on airway monitoring, fluid resuscitation, and antibiotic therapy. Antibiotic coverage should be broad until cultures have resulted and should be directed at the most common organisms. Hoffman and colleagues[34] reported a case series with results showing *Streptococcus* isolated from 72% (*Streptococcus pyogenes* 41%) of cultures, *Staphylococcus aureus* 13%, *Candida albicans* 6%, *H influenzae* 3%, *Fusobacterium* spp 3%, and *Abiotrophia* spp 3%.

Complications from RPA are potentially disastrous. The complication rate in a study looking at the KIDS' Inpatient Database was 4.8% (2.8% respiratory failure, 1.6% sepsis).[38] Notably, children have fewer instances of descending mediastinitis.[33]

LEMIERRE SYNDROME

Lemierre syndrome is typically caused by the anaerobic, gram-negative *Fusobacterium necrophorum*. Lemierre syndrome classically follows an episode of pharyngitis and/or PTA, which subsequently leads to septic thrombophlebitis of the ipsilateral internal jugular vein. This can ultimately lead to sepsis and septic emboli. In modern usage, the term Lemierre syndrome is often used for all infections with *Fusobacterium necrophorum* resulting from an origin not only in the oropharynx but also the face, ears, mastoid, and teeth. Lemierre syndrome is most commonly precipitated by otitis media in the pediatric populations, tonsillitis or PTA in young adults, and dental infections in adults.[40]

The classic symptoms for Lemierre syndrome are oropharyngeal pain, fever, neck swelling, pulmonary symptoms, and arthralgias.[41] Metastatic abscesses are common and result from septic emboli from the internal jugular vein thrombophlebitis.[42] Lungs are involved in up to 85% of cases and manifest as bilateral necrotic infiltrates, pleural effusions, empyema, or pulmonary abscesses. Joint involvement is seen up to 26% of the time, with sterile effusions or suppurative arthritis being most common. More rare complications include intraabdominal abscesses, hepatic abscesses, osteomyelitis, endocarditis, and meningitis.[41]

Treatment is primarily medical management with IV fluid resuscitation and IV antibiotics. Despite advances in detection and treatment, mortality for Lemierre syndrome remains as high as 17%.[41] *Fusobacterium necrophorum* is frequently reported to be susceptible to penicillin, cephalosporins, metronidazole, clindamycin, tetracyclines, and chloramphenicol.[43] Monotherapy with metronidazole is not recommended owing to the common co-occurrence of resistant organisms.[44] A reasonable initial treatment is penicillin G at 1.2 to 3.0 g 4 times daily (children, 24–60 mg/kg 4 times daily) and IV metronidazole 500 mg 3 times daily (children, 10–15 mg/kg 3 times daily). Alternatively, monotherapy with IV clindamycin at 0.6 to 0.9 g 3 times daily (children, 10 mg/kg 3 times daily) can be used.[40] Surgical treatment is often necessary to drain an empyema, debride necrotic tissue,[45] or treat mediastinitis.[46] Anticoagulation is not advised in Lemierre syndrome because it is thought to increase the likelihood of causing septic emboli.

ACUTE SUPPURATIVE PAROTITIS

Acute suppurative parotitis (ASP) occurs most commonly in children younger than 2 months of age or in geriatric patients with systemic illness or recent surgical procedures. ASP can present as a single episode or with multiple recurrences. Some of the most common factors associated with ASP are found in **Box 1**. Noninfectious causes of parotid swelling should also be considered, including collagen-vascular disease,

---

Box 1
Factors associated with acute suppurative parotitis

Infectious
    Oral infection (eg, dental infection)

Noninfectious
    Medications (eg, tranquilizers, antihistamines, diuretics)
    Dehydration
    Malnutrition
    Immunosuppression
    Neoplasm of oral cavity
    Tracheotomy
    Sialectasis
    Ductal obstruction

cystic fibrosis, alcoholism, diabetes, gout, uremia, sarcoidosis, sialolithiasis, and tumors. The list of differential diagnoses of nonparotid swelling mimicking ASP includes lymphoma, lymphangitis, cervical adenitis, external otitis, and dental abscess.[47]

The typical presentation of patients with ASP is sudden onset of warm, tender, red swelling of the cheek, usually unilateral, extending to the angle of the mandible (**Fig. 3**). The parotid orifice is erythematous and pus may be draining or expressed with gentle pressure on the duct. The presence of purulent drainage differentiates bacterial parotitis from viral causes such as mumps, HIV, Epstein-Barr virus, and influenza.[47]

Treatment of acute bacterial parotitis is with IV antibiotics and adequate parenteral hydration. Historically, the most common pathogen in ASP has been *Staphylococcus aureus* (over 80% of cases), with streptococci and gram-negative rods such as *Escherichia coli* also being frequently isolated. Typically, a penicillinase-resistant penicillin such as nafcillin is adequate.[48] However, the incidence of ASP caused by anaerobes is increasing. Some investigators suggest broad-spectrum antibiotics covering aerobic and anaerobic organisms be started in ASP. Clindamycin, cefoxitin, imipenem, meropenem, or metronidazole and a macrolide will provide adequate coverage if an anaerobic infection is suspected. Needle aspiration of the parotid gland is the best method to determine the causative organism.[47]

When a parotid abscess has formed, surgical drainage is indicated. Physical examination findings such as fluctuance typically do not appear until late in the course. Imaging with ultrasound or CT scan is useful to detect abscess formation. Worsening of clinical course progressing to sepsis is also an indication for surgical drainage.[47]

DESCENDING NECROTIZING MEDIASTINITIS

Descending necrotizing mediastinitis (DNM) is an acute, rapidly progressive polymicrobial infection of the mediastinum with reported mortality rates ranging from 30% to 50%.[49] From the neck to the mediastinum, there are 3 potential major pathways for infection to spread along the fascial spaces in DNM: (1) the pretracheal route to the anterior mediastinum, (2) the lateral pharyngeal route to the middle mediastinum,

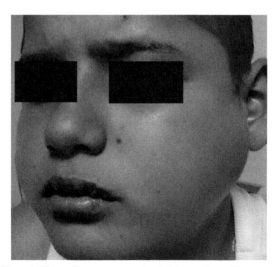

Fig. 3. Parotitis. (*From* Wikimedia commons. Available at: https://commons.wikimedia.org/wiki/File:Parotiditis_(Parotitis;_Mumps).JPG. Accessed June 2, 2018.)

and (3) the retropharyngeal route to the posterior mediastinum. Posterior to the retropharyngeal space is the danger space. The alar fascia separates the 2 spaces. The importance of the danger space, and the source for its sinister moniker, is that it extends from the skull base to the level of the diaphragm, providing a pathway into the posterior mediastinum and pleural spaces from the head and neck. Infection in the danger space most commonly occurs when an abscess in the retropharyngeal space ruptures through the alar fascia.[50]

DNM results from oropharyngeal abscesses with resultant severe cervical infection, most commonly odontogenic, peritonsillar, or retropharyngeal infections.[51] Gravity, respiration, and negative intrathoracic pressure are believed to accelerate intrathoracic spread.[52] Acute mediastinitis not from an oropharyngeal source is frequently caused by iatrogenic oropharyngeal perforation, cervical trauma, epiglottitis, parotitis, sinusitis, sternoclavicular joint infections, and IV drug use. Surgical procedures involving lymph node biopsy in the neck, thyroidectomy, tracheostomy, and mediastinoscopy rarely lead to mediastinitis.[51]

Onset of symptoms is acute and involves fever, chest pain, dysphagia, and respiratory distress. Fortunately, the inciting infection is usually readily apparent because the patient will complain of neck pain, dysphagia, and/or odynophagia. Chest radiographs may demonstrate diffuse mediastinal widening and gas bubbles, or a fluid level suggesting a mediastinal abscess. Chest CT scan is the test of choice in diagnosis of DNM. It will reveal the presence of mediastinal fluid collection, extraluminal gas, pericardial and pleural effusions, and soft tissue edema.[51] Cervical CT scan is also required because it will often reveal the origin of the infection.[53] Estrera and colleagues[54] described diagnostic criteria for DNM (**Box 2**).

Broad-spectrum antibiotics such as piperacillin-tazobactam should be initiated. DNM is typically polymicrobial, often involving usual oral flora. Anaerobes generally outnumber aerobes in DNM. The organisms most commonly implicated include *Prevotella*, *Peptostreptococcus*, *Fusobacterium*, *Veillonella*, *Actinomyces*, and oral *Streptococcus*.[49]

Surgical drainage is the definitive treatment and involvement of a thoracic surgeon should occur immediately. Approaches to drainage differ and can be limited to cervical approach only or include a thoracotomy after cervical approach to drainage.[51]

PREVERTEBRAL SPACE INFECTIONS

Prevertebral space infections can be especially challenging to detect. The prevertebral space lies posterior to the danger space and is bordered anteriorly by the prevertebral fascia and posteriorly by the vertebral bodies and deep cervical musculature.

Box 2
Diagnostic criteria for descending necrotizing mediastinitis

1. Evidence of severe oropharyngeal infection

2. Radiologic findings of mediastinitis

3. Findings of necrotizing mediastinitis at operation and/or postmortem

4. Establishment of relationship between oropharyngeal infection and necrotizing mediastinal process

Data from Estrera AS, Landay MJ, Grisham JM, et al. Descending necrotizing mediastinitis. Surg Gynecol Obstet 1983;157(6):545–52.

The danger space allows infections to track downward to the level of the mediastinum. This can result in mediastinitis, empyema, and sepsis. The prevertebral space extends down the entire length of the vertebral column to the coccyx and is contiguous with the psoas sheath.[55] Dense fibrous attachments between the prevertebral fascia and deep cervical muscles tend to contain prevertebral infections, preventing longitudinal spread. Sources of prevertebral space infections include posterior pharyngeal trauma, secondary spread from Pott abscesses, and extension from retropharyngeal and danger space infections, as well as cervical and thoracic spine osteomyelitis and discitis.[55]

The presentation of infections of the prevertebral space depends on the degree of spinal cord compression and neurologic dysfunction. The diagnosis of prevertebral abscesses is often difficult and nearly half of cases are initially misdiagnosed.[56] Roughly 75% of patients experience back or neck pain, 50% present with fever, and 33% have neurologic deficits ranging in severity from nerve root pain to paralysis. Irreversible paralysis occurs in 4% to 22% of patients.[57]

MRI is the diagnostic test of choice for prevertebral space infections to assess involvement of the epidural space or spinal cord.[58] Broad-spectrum IV antibiotics are the mainstay of treatment, along with spine surgery consultation. Surgical approach is typically via an external cervical approach rather than intraoral to limit the potential for a persistent draining fistula in the posterior pharynx.[59] The most common pathogens implicated in prevertebral space infections are *Staphylococcus aureus*, oral anaerobes, and enteric gram-negative rods. Recent reports have found that early surgical intervention is associated with lower morbidity and mortality than medical therapy alone.[60]

SUMMARY

Soft tissue infections of the neck range from the common (eg, pharyngitis) to the unusual and life-threatening (eg, DNM). ED providers should appreciate the complexity of neck anatomy and have a diagnostic approach to patients with concerning symptoms and signs of the neck, such as dysphagia or odynophagia, pain, erythema, and swelling. Some neck infections require immediate surgical consultation and some necessitate antibiotics. Airway monitoring may also be a critical aspect of the emergency care of these infections.

REFERENCES

1. Christian JM. Odontogenic infections. Cummings otolaryngology - head and neck surgery. 5th edition. Amsterdam, Netherlands: Elsevier Health Sciences; 2010. p. 177–90.
2. Alcaide ML, Bisno AL. Pharyngitis and epiglottitis. Infect Dis Clin North Am 2007; 21(3):847–8.
3. Salkind AR. Economic burden of GAS pharyngitis substantial. Pharmacoeconomics 2008;11(4):621–7.
4. Shulman ST, Bisno AL, Clegg HW, et al. Clinical practice guideline for the diagnosis and management of group A streptococcal pharyngitis: 2012 update by the Infectious Diseases Society of America. Clin Infect Dis 2012;55(10):1279–82.
5. Lean WL, Arnup S, Danchin M, et al. Rapid diagnostic tests for group a streptococcal pharyngitis: meta-analysis. Pediatrics 2014;134(4):771–81.
6. Demuri GP, Wald ER. The group A streptococcal carrier state reviewed: still an enigma. J Pediatric Infect Dis Soc 2014;3(4):336–42.

7. Centor R, Witherspoon J, Dalton H, et al. The diagnosis of strep throat in adults in the emergency room. Med Decis Making 1981;1:239–46.

8. Cooper RJ, Hoffman JR, Bartlett JG, et al. Principles of appropriate antibiotic use for acute pharyngitis in adults: background. Ann Intern Med 2001;134(6):509–17.

9. Bulloch B, Kabani A, Tenenbein M. Oral dexamethasone for the treatment of pain in children with acute pharyngitis: a randomized, double-blind, placebo-controlled trial. Ann Emerg Med 2003;41(5):601–8.

10. Korb K, Scherer M, Chenot JF. Steroids as adjuvant therapy for acute pharyngitis in ambulatory patients: a systematic review. Ann Fam Med 2010;8(1):58–63.

11. Marvez-Valls EG, Stuckey A, Ernst AA. A randomized clinical trial of oral versus intramuscular delivery of steroids in acute exudative pharyngitis. Acad Emerg Med 2002;9(1):9–14.

12. Frantz TD, Rasgon BM. Acute epiglottitis: changing epidemiologic patterns. Otolaryngol Head Neck Surg 1993;109(3 Pt 1):457–60.

13. Cherry J, Demmler-Harrison GJ, Hotez PJ, et al. Feigin and Cherry's textbook of pediatric infectious diseases. Philadelphia (PA): Saunders W.B.; 2018.

14. Lee SH, Yun SJ, Kim DH, et al. Do we need a change in ED diagnostic strategy for adult acute epiglottitis? Am J Emerg Med 2017;35(10):1519–24.

15. Ko DR, Chung YE, Park I, et al. Use of bedside sonography for diagnosing acute epiglottitis in the emergency department: a preliminary study. J Ultrasound Med 2012;31(1):19–22.

16. Werner SL, Jones RA, Emerman CL. Sonographic assessment of the epiglottis. Acad Emerg Med 2004;11(12):1358–60.

17. Gilbert DN, Chambers HF, Eliopoulos GM, et al. Sanford guide to antimicrobial therapy 2017. Sperryville (VA): Antimicrobial Therapy, Inc.; 2017.

18. Shah RK, Roberson DW, Jones DT. Epiglottitis in the *Hemophilus influenzae* type B vaccine era: changing trends. Laryngoscope 2004;114(3):557–60.

19. Stage J, Bonding P. Peritonsillar abscess with parapharyngeal involvement: incidence and treatment. Clin Otolaryngol Allied Sci 1987;12(1):1–5.

20. Powell J, Wilson J. An evidence-based review of peritonsillar abscess. Clin Otolaryngol 2012;37(2):136–45.

21. Klug TE. Incidence and microbiology of peritonsillar abscess: the influence of season, age, and gender. Eur J Clin Microbiol Infect Dis 2014;33(7):1163–7.

22. Powell EL, Powell J, Samuel JR, et al. A review of the pathogenesis of adult peritonsillar abscess: time for a re-evaluation. J Antimicrob Chemother 2013;68(9):1941–50.

23. Plum AW, Mortelliti AJ, Walsh RE. Microbial flora and antibiotic resistance in peritonsillar abscesses in upstate New York. Ann Otol Rhinol Laryngol 2015;124(11):875–80.

24. Kieff DA, Bhattacharyya N, Siegel NS, et al. Selection of antibiotics after incision and drainage of peritonsillar abscesses. Otolaryngol Head Neck Surg 1999;120(1):57–61.

25. Chau JKM, Seikaly HR, Harris JR, et al. Corticosteroids in peritonsillar abscess treatment: a blinded placebo-controlled clinical trial. Laryngoscope 2013;124(1):97–103.

26. Ozbek C, Aygenc E, Tuna EU, et al. Use of steroids in the treatment of peritonsillar abscess. J Laryngol Otol 2004;118(6):439–42.

27. Chang BA, Thamboo A, Burton MJ, et al. Needle aspiration versus incision and drainage for the treatment of peritonsillar abscess. Cochrane Database Syst Rev 2016;(12):CD006287.

28. Saifeldeen K. Ludwigs angina. Emerg Med J 2004;21(2):242–3.

29. Kao S, Girn J, Jo C, et al. Ludwig's angina. In: Bagheri SC, editor. Clinical review of oral and maxillofacial surgery. 2nd edition. Miami (FL): Elsevier Health Sciences; 2014. p. 95–118.
30. Botha A, Jacobs F, Postma C. Retrospective analysis of etiology and comorbid diseases associated with Ludwig's Angina. Ann Maxillofac Surg 2015;5(2): 168–73.
31. Busch RF, Shah D. Ludwig's angina: improved treatment. Otolaryngol Head Neck Surg 1997;117:S172–5.
32. Freund B, Timon C. Ludwig's angina: a place for steroid therapy in its management. Oral Health 1992;82(5):23–5.
33. Kirse DJ, Roberson DW. Surgical management of retropharyngeal space infections in children. Laryngoscope 2001;111(8):1413–22.
34. Hoffmann C, Pierrot S, Contencin P, et al. Retropharyngeal infections in children. Treatment strategies and outcomes. Int J Pediatr Otorhinolaryngol 2011;75(9): 1099–103.
35. Wetmore RF, Mahboubi S, Soyupak SK. Computed tomography in the evaluation of pediatric neck infections. Otolaryngol Head Neck Surg 1998;119(6):624–7.
36. Lalakea ML, Messner AH. Retropharyngeal abscess management in children: current practices. Otolaryngol Head Neck Surg 1999;121(4):398–405.
37. Collins B, Stoner JA, Digoy GP. Benefits of ultrasound vs. computed tomography in the diagnosis of pediatric lateral neck abscesses. Int J Pediatr Otorhinolaryngol 2014;78(3):423–6.
38. Adil E, Tarshish Y, Roberson D, et al. The public health impact of pediatric deep neck space infections. Otolaryngol Head Neck Surg 2015;153(6):1036–41.
39. Cheng J, Elden L. Children with deep space neck infections: our experience with 178 children. Otolaryngol Head Neck Surg 2013;148(6):1037–42.
40. Hagelskjaer Kristensen L, Prag J. Human necrobacillosis, with emphasis on Lemierre's syndrome. Clin Infect Dis 2000;31(2):524–32.
41. Leugers CM, Clover R. Lemierre syndrome: postanginal sepsis. J Am Board Fam Pract 1995;8(5):384–91.
42. Seidenfeld SM, Sutker WL, Luby JP. *Fusobacterium necrophorum* septicemia following oropharyngeal infection. JAMA 1982;248(11):1348–50.
43. Lechtenberg KF, Nagaraja TG, Chengappa MM. Antimicrobial susceptibility of *Fusobacterium necrophorum* isolated from bovine hepatic abscesses. Am J Vet Res 1998;59(1):44–7.
44. Bartlett JG. Anaerobic bacterial infections of the lung and pleural space. Clin Infect Dis 1993;16(Suppl 4):S248–55.
45. Civen R, Jousimies-Somer H, Marina M, et al. A retrospective review of cases of anaerobic empyema and update of bacteriology. Clin Infect Dis 1995;20(Suppl 2):S224–9.
46. Marty-Ane CH, Alauzen M, Alric P, et al. Descending necrotizing mediastinitis. Advantage of mediastinal drainage with thoracotomy. J Thorac Cardiovasc Surg 1994;107(1):55–61.
47. Brook I. Acute bacterial suppurative parotitis: microbiology and management. J Craniofac Surg 2003;14(1):37–40.
48. Fattahi TT, Lyu PE, Van Sickels JE. Management of acute suppurative parotitis. J Oral Maxillofac Surg 2002;60(4):446–8.
49. Pinto A, Scaglione M, Scuderi MG, et al. Infections of the neck leading to descending necrotizing mediastinitis: role of multi-detector row computed tomography. Eur J Radiol 2008;65(3):389–94.

50. Smith JK, Armao DM, Specter BB, et al. Danger space infection: infection of the neck leading to descending necrotizing mediastinitis. Emerg Radiol 1999;6(3): 129–32.
51. Athanassiadi KA. Infections of the mediastinum. Thorac Surg Clin 2009;19(1): 37–45.
52. Marty-Ané C-H, Berthet J-P, Alric P, et al. Management of descending necrotizing mediastinitis: an aggressive treatment for an aggressive disease. Ann Thorac Surg 1999;68(1):212–7.
53. Brunelli A, Sabbatini A, Catalini G, et al. Descending necrotizing mediastinitis. Surgical drainage and tracheostomy. Arch Otolaryngol Head Neck Surg 1996; 122(12):1326–9.
54. Estrera AS, Landay MJ, Grisham JM, et al. Descending necrotizing mediastinitis. Surg Gynecol Obstet 1983;157(6):545–52.
55. Grewal S, Hocking G, Wildsmith JA. Epidural abscesses. Br J Anaesth 2006; 96(3):292–302.
56. Davis DP, Wold RM, Patel RJ, et al. The clinical presentation and impact of diagnostic delays on emergency department patients with spinal epidural abscess. J Emerg Med 2004;26(3):285–91.
57. Reihsaus E, Waldbaur H, Seeling W. Spinal epidural abscess: a meta-analysis of 915 patients. Neurosurg Rev 2000;23(4):175–204.
58. Stäbler A, Reiser MF. Imaging of spinal infection. Radiol Clin North Am 2001; 39(1):115–35.
59. Vieira F, Allen SM, Stocks RM, et al. Deep neck infection. Otolaryngol Clin North Am 2008;41(3):459–83.
60. Curry WT Jr, Hoh BL, Amin-Hanjani S, et al. Spinal epidural abscess: clinical presentation, management, and outcome. Surg Neurol 2005;63(4):364–71.

Tracheostomy Emergencies

Laura J. Bontempo, MD, MEd*, Sara L. Manning, MD

KEYWORDS

- Tracheostomy • Airway • Decannulation • Obstruction
- Tracheoinnominate artery fistula • Tracheal stenosis

KEY POINTS

- Replacement of a decannulated tracheostomy fewer than 7 days old should be attempted only under direct visualization.
- A completely obstructed tracheostomy tube must be removed to maintain airway patency.
- All tracheostomy bleeding should be considered a sentinel bleed and the source must be identified, even if the bleeding resolves.
- Chronic and subacute tracheostomy complications can present months to years after placement or decannulation.

INTRODUCTION

More than 110,000 tracheostomies are placed annually in the United States.[1] The overall complication incidence is 40% to 50%. Thankfully, the vast majority of these complications are minor. One percent of tracheostomy patients, however, will suffer a catastrophic tracheostomy-related complication. Of those patients, up to half will die. It is, therefore, incumbent for the emergency provider to be able to recognize the signs and symptoms of tracheostomy-related emergencies and provide initial stabilization and, potentially, life-saving interventions.

Tracheostomy-related complications are generally grouped by their peak incidence of occurrence.[2,3] Intraoperative complications, including hemorrhage, air embolism, and damage to the trachea, are not within the treatment domain of the emergency physician and will not be discussed here. Intermediate (early postoperative) complications include hemorrhage, tube decannulation, extratracheal air (subcutaneous emphysema, pneumothorax, pneumomediastinum), and infection. Late postoperative complications include hemorrhage, tracheal stenosis, tube decannulation, and fistula formation.[2,4] The delineation between intermediate and late complications is variable;

Disclosure Statement: The authors have no financial interests to disclose.
Department of Emergency Medicine, University of Maryland School of Medicine, 110 South Paca Street, 6th Floor, Suite 200, Baltimore, MD 21201, USA
* Corresponding author.
E-mail address: lbontempo@som.umaryland.edu

Emerg Med Clin N Am 37 (2019) 109–119
https://doi.org/10.1016/j.emc.2018.09.010
0733-8627/19/© 2018 Elsevier Inc. All rights reserved.

however, the Agency for Healthcare Research and Quality reported that tracheostomies have the fifth-highest 30-day readmission rate for procedures performed during the index stay. Nearly 1 in 4 patients with tracheostomy will require hospital admission within 30 days of having their tracheostomy placed.[5] More than 90% of catastrophic complications occur more than 1 week after tracheostomy placement.[6]

For the purposes of emergency management, tracheostomy complications are grouped into emergent life-threatening complications and urgent complications. Emergent life-threatening complications include tube decannulation, tube obstruction, and hemorrhage. Urgent subacute complications include tracheoesophageal fistula formation, tracheal stenosis, infection, and tracheocutaneous fistula formation.

The management of both emergent and urgent tracheostomy complications may be further complicated by the underlying condition of the patient who originally necessitated the placement of the tracheostomy. Indications for tracheostomy placement include upper respiratory tract obstruction, prolonged ventilation, copious secretions, severe obstructive sleep apnea, and head/neck surgery.[3] Such comorbid conditions must be considered when making management decisions.

ANATOMY

Tracheostomies are placed using a percutaneous dilational approach or open surgical approach. With either approach, the goal is to create an opening into the trachea through the anterior neck where the tracheal mucosa is brought into continuity with the skin.[7] The complication rate between the 2 techniques is similar.[8] The indications for performing a tracheostomy are upper airway obstruction, control of secretions, the necessity of long-term ventilation, and the necessity for long-term airway protection.[9,10]

Using either technique, tracheostomies are generally placed between the second and third tracheal rings.[11] Higher incisions increase the risk of laryngeal injury and lower incisions increase the risk of decannulation and vessel injury.[7]

EMERGENT LIFE-THREATENING COMPLICATIONS
Tracheostomy Decannulation

Inadvertent tracheostomy tube decannulation can occur at any time following tracheostomy placement. The reported incidence of tracheostomy displacement varies widely. The literature reports rates between 0.35% and 15%.[2,12,13] It is the second most frequent life-threatening early pediatric tracheostomy complication,[14] and in the critical care setting, 50% of airway-related deaths were associated with tracheostomy displacement.[15] Many decannulations may be handled by the patient or caregiver without seeking further care, so the incidence may be higher than reported. Decannulations within the first week of placement are most concerning because of the lack of mature stoma formation and a narrower tracheocutaneous tract, which increases the risk of airway loss.[16]

Risk factors for accidental tracheostomy decannulation include mental status change, traumatic brain injury, increased secretions, recent tracheostomy change, increased neck thickness, and pediatric age.[2,14,16] Tracheostomies placed using a percutaneous technique are at higher risk for decannulation than those placed using an open surgical approach.[3]

When a patient presents to the Emergency Department (ED) with a displaced tracheostomy tube, 2 key pieces of information must be obtained. First, how long ago was the tracheostomy placed, and second, how long before presentation did the tracheostomy become decannulated. The patient may present with the tracheostomy completely displaced from the stoma or with the tracheostomy partially displaced with the tip present in the soft tissue of the neck. When decannulation occurs, replacement without delay is indicated. Even a mature stoma may significantly narrow over the course of hours, making delayed recannulation more challenging and necessitating the use of a smaller tracheostomy tube during replacement.[17]

Replacement of a dislodged tracheostomy within the first week of placement should be attempted only with direct visualization via fiberoptic endoscopy to reduce the risk of creating a false passage into the soft tissue of the neck.[3,17] If fiberoptic visualization is unavailable or is unsuccessful, then oral intubation may be necessary to secure the airway and ventilate the patient (**Fig. 1**). For tracheostomies placed more than 7 days before dislodgement, a new tracheostomy tube may be inserted through the stoma with placement then confirmed by fiberoptic visualization.

Regardless of the age of the tracheostomy, if resistance is met, a smaller tracheostomy tube should be selected and insertion reattempted. If recannulating is unsuccessful, bag-valve ventilation and oral intubation may be necessary if the patient fails to oxygenate or ventilate.[3,17,18] If a replacement tracheostomy tube is not readily available, an analogous size endotracheal tube may be inserted through the stoma until a tracheostomy tube can be obtained.[18]

Following recannulation, low-volume, gentle bag-valve ventilation can be used to assist ventilation.[15] If subcutaneous emphysema develops, tracheostomy placement must be evaluated through direct visualization due to possible false passage with placement of the tracheostomy tube into the paratracheal soft tissue of the

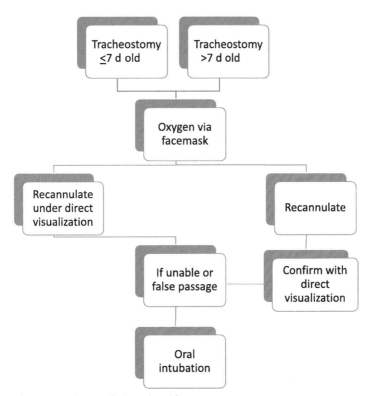

Fig. 1. Tracheostomy decannulation algorithm.

neck.[19,20] If proper placement is confirmed, the trachea must be subsequently evaluated for injury. Once recannulated, continuous capnometry is used to monitor ventilation.

Tracheostomy Obstruction

Obstruction of the lumen of a tracheostomy tube can result from dried secretions, mucous plugs, clotted blood, partial tube displacement, impingement by the posterior tracheal wall, granulation tissue buildup, or displacement of the tracheostomy into a false lumen. It can occur at any time and is the leading cause of tracheostomy-related death in pediatric patients.[6] Risk factors for obstruction include small tracheostomy tube size, single cannula tracheostomy tube, and poor tracheostomy care.[3,18]

Management of tracheotomy obstruction requires a stepwise approach (**Fig. 2**). An initial simple step is to remove anything potentially obstructing the external end of the tracheostomy lumen, such as a speaking valve, obturator, decannulation cap, bandages, or humidifying devices.[15] Removal of the inner cannula of a double-cannula tracheostomy and suctioning of single or double-cannula tracheostomies are the next steps when obstruction is suspected and will relieve most obstructions.[3,18]

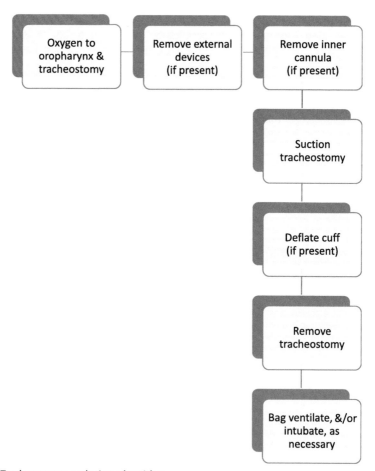

Fig. 2. Tracheostomy occlusion algorithm.

If a suction catheter can be passed through the entire length of the tracheostomy into the native trachea, a complete obstruction is not present. The patient's ventilation can be assisted with positive pressure as necessary to improve ventilation and oxygenation. If a suction catheter cannot be passed, a complete obstruction of the tracheostomy tube is present. Stiff instruments, such as gum-elastic bougies and tube changers, are not recommended to assess patency because they do not allow for removal of secretions and can create a false passage if the tracheostomy is obstructed due to partial or complete displacement.[15]

If the tracheostomy tube is cuffed, the cuff must be deflated to allow for airflow around the tracheostomy tube because flow through the tracheostomy tube lumen is occluded. If the obstruction is relieved by other means or if a new tracheostomy is placed, the balloon will need to be inflated to provide effective positive pressure ventilation.

When, despite these measures, a patient continues to be distressed from airway obstruction, the tracheostomy tube must be removed. Although removing the artificial airway may seem counterintuitive in a distressed patient, a nonfunctioning tracheostomy offers no benefit to the patient. Following removal, ensure that the patient is receiving high-flow oxygen via both face and tracheostomy stoma. If the obstruction is relieved and the patient is ventilating, as monitored by capnometry, it is not necessary to emergently reinsert an airway.[15]

Following tracheostomy removal, if bag-valve-mask ventilatory assistance is used, it is necessary to remember that the patient has 2 airway openings (tracheostomy and oro-nasopharynx). If the patient is ventilated via the mouth, the tracheal stoma must be occluded with gauze (**Fig. 3**). If the patient is ventilated via the tracheal stoma, the oral and nasal pharynx must be occluded. To generate airway positive pressure when ventilating, a pediatric face mask or laryngeal-mask airway can be placed over the stoma (**Fig. 4**).[15] If effective oxygenation and ventilation is not achieved with bag-valve maneuvers, intubation should be attempted. If intubating by the oropharynx, the endotracheal tube must be advanced beyond the stoma to generate positive pressure in the lower airway after the balloon is inflated. If the tracheostomy is more than a week old or if oral intubation is anticipated to be difficult, intubation of the stoma can be attempted. A smaller tracheostomy tube or endotracheal tube can be placed

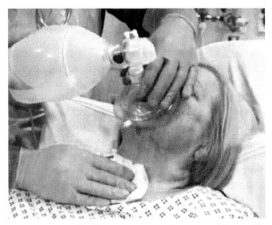

Fig. 3. Occluding the ostomy to facilitate oro-nasopharyngeal bag-valve-mask ventilation. (*Courtesy of* National Tracheostomy Safety Project; with permission.)

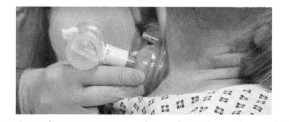

Fig. 4. Ventilating via tracheostomy stoma with a pediatric bag-valve-mask. (*Courtesy of* National Tracheostomy Safety Project; with permission.)

directly into the stoma. Guided placement using a fiberoptic scope, Bougie, or tube exchange catheter is preferred.[15]

When the obstruction is partially or completely relieved after any step in the algorithm, the patient's ventilation should be monitored with continuous capnometry and pulse-oximetry and assisted with positive pressure ventilation as the clinical situation necessitates.

Hemorrhage

Tracheostomy bleeding complicates up to 5% of tracheostomies and ranges from minor to life-threatening. Bleeding within the first 48 hours after placement is usually related to operative issues, including inadvertent vein puncture, suctioning, and infection.[21] Beyond 48 hours, the most critical and feared hemorrhagic complication is the development of a tracheo-innominate artery (TIAF) fistula. This is a direct connection between the native trachea and the innominate artery branch of the aorta. The incidence of TIAF is approximately 0.7% of patients with tracheostomy and the mortality is more than 90%.[2,21,22] Nearly 75% of TIAF bleeds will occur within 3 weeks following tracheostomy placement but may occur at any time.[21–23]

Up to 50% of TIAF bleeds will have a sentinel event, such as tracheostomy site bleeding, hemoptysis, or blood seen with tracheal suctioning.[21] Therefore, any tracheostomy-related hemorrhage, especially occurring within 3 weeks of placement, must be considered a TIAF bleed until proven otherwise. Diagnostic options include bronchoscopy, computed tomography or traditional angiography, or local exploration.[18,24]

The innominate artery crosses anterior to the trachea, typically at the level of the ninth tracheal ring; however, there is significant anatomic variation and the innominate artery may cross the trachea superior enough to be anterior to a tracheostomy tube. Pressure on the anterior tracheal wall results in mucosal ischemia and can lead to fistula formation with the posterior wall of the innominate artery. Risk factors include a cuffed tracheostomy tube, low tracheostomy placement, high cuff pressure, high-riding innominate artery, excessive neck movement, and tracheostomy infection.[23,25]

If catastrophic tracheostomy bleeding occurs, a TIAF should be assumed and immediate resuscitative measures undertaken while attempts to temporize the bleeding and facilitate operative repair are made (**Fig. 5**). Initial intervention attempts include external compression of the innominate artery by applying pressure posteriorly at the sternal notch, and internal compression through overinflation of the tracheostomy balloon with up to 50 mL of air. These interventions are reported to be successful as a temporizing measure 85% of the time.[23] If a cuffed tracheostomy tube is not present or overinflation has failed to control the bleeding, the tracheostomy tube can be removed and the airway secured via oral or stomal intubation with an endotracheal

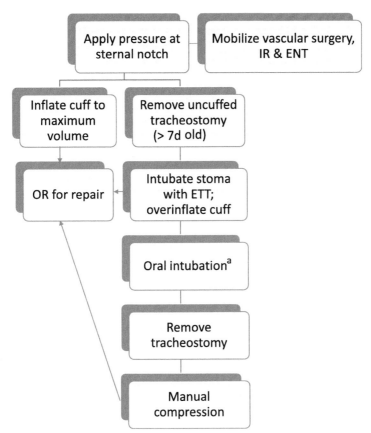

Fig. 5. Large-volume tracheostomy hemorrhage algorithm. ENT, otolaryngology; ETT, endotracheal tube; IR, interventional radiology; OR, operating room. [a] Advance balloon distal to tracheostomy then inflate; may require concurrent tracheostomy removal.

tube whose cuff is then overinflated with up to 50 mL of air. If this also proves to be unsuccessful, an oral endotracheal tube can be advanced beyond the stoma to secure the airway with the addition of a finger inserted into the tracheostomy for digital compression of the innominate artery anteriorly against the manubrium.[26] Digital compression must be maintained until definitive repair is undertaken.

These maneuvers are all performed in an attempt to decrease the amount of blood loss while getting the patient to the operating room or interventional radiology suite for definitive management.[21]

URGENT COMPLICATIONS
Tracheoesophageal Fistula

A tracheoesophageal fistula (TEF) is a communication between the posterior wall of the trachea and the anterior wall of the esophagus. Prolonged pressure on the posterior membranous wall of the trachea from a tracheostomy balloon results in ischemic necrosis, tissue breakdown, and subsequent fistula formation.[27] Risk factors include high airway pressures, prolonged presence of a cuffed tracheostomy tube, high cuff pressures, excessive tracheostomy movement, steroid use, type 1 diabetes mellitus, chronic hypoxia, poor nutritional status, hypotension, anemia, sepsis, the presence of a nasogastric tube, and gastro-esophageal reflux disease (GERD).[27,28]

TEFs may manifest as persistent tracheal air leaks, abdominal distention (from air entering the digestive tract), pulmonary aspiration injury, cough with swallowing, copious bronchopulmonary secretions, and respiratory distress. In patients with tracheostomy, the TEF is generally located 1 to 2 cm distal to the tracheal stoma at the level of the balloon and can be large, measuring 4 to 5 cm. Diagnosis is made by bronchoscopy or, if not available, esophagram.

Emergency management includes stopping contamination of the airway through tracheal suctioning, discontinuation of oral feeding, and elevation of the patient's head to 45°. If a gastric tube is present, it should be used to drain the contents of the stomach. However, if a nasogastric tube is in place, it should be removed to prevent pressure necrosis and worsening of the fistula.[27] Additionally, any suppurative complications, such as pneumonia, should be treated.

Long-term treatment consists of conservative management with adjustment of the tracheostomy balloon to a more distal position and nutrition via jejunostomy tube, minimally invasive treatment with tracheal and esophageal stents, or surgery.[27]

Tracheal Stenosis

Tracheal stenosis is common after prolonged intubation or tracheostomy, with most patients experiencing some degree of tracheal narrowing. However, only 3% to 12% of cases require any intervention and very few of those patients experience critical stenosis requiring urgent intervention.[2,29,30] Stenosis occurs secondary to granulation tissue and fibrosis of peristomal and tracheal tissues. After granulation tissue forms, it eventually becomes covered with epithelial tissue.[3]

Trauma to the trachea either from injury during the procedure itself or ischemia from balloon over inflation leads to tracheal inflammation and ulceration. Other risk factors include surgical site infection, GERD, obesity, and hypotension.[29,30] Tracheal stenosis frequently occurs at the site of the stoma, the level of the tracheostomy tube tip, the site of the balloon, or in a suprastomal position. Stenosis will not cause symptoms until the diameter of the tracheal lumen is reduced by more than 50%.[29,30] Early symptoms include difficulty clearing secretions, cough, and exertional dyspnea. Dyspnea at rest and stridor are associated with a tracheal diameter of ≤ 5 mm.[29] Tracheal stenosis can occur while a patient is still mechanically ventilated or years after decannulation, but most will present within 2 months of decannulation.[3]

Stenosis can make tube exchanges difficult due to narrowing of the space and bleeding risk. Early stenosis with exposed granulation tissue without overlying epithelium can bleed easily with minor trauma.[29] Stenosis can be treated with dilation, excision with end-to-end anastomosis, or laser excision of granulation or fibrous tissues.[3,30]

Infection

Tracheostomy is considered a "clean-contaminated" procedure due to the entrance of the upper aerodigestive tract. Bacterial colonization of the skin and aerodigestive tract combined with the rich environment of blood and secretions at the surgical site place patients at risk of surgical site infection. Strict wound care with frequent dressing changes is the cornerstone of preventing infection after tracheostomy. Common early infections include cellulitis and tracheitis.[2] These infections frequently occur early in the postoperative course and are more commonly observed after open versus percutaneous tracheostomy.[3] Most early infections are minor, but severe infections, including mediastinitis and necrotizing fasciitis, are possible.[31] Delayed presentations of serious infections have been observed, most notably osteomyelitis and septic arthritis of the sternoclavicular joint.[32]

The presence of a tracheostomy tube, especially a cuffed tube, disrupts swallowing, thus increasing the risk of aspiration. An overinflated tube cuff can compress the esophagus, leading to aspiration. This aspiration is often asymptomatic or silent and therefore unrecognized by patients and caregivers.[29] Aspiration of infected secretions can result in pneumonia or lung abscesses. These infections are most commonly attributed to *Staphylococcus aureus, Pseudomonas,* and mixed flora.[2]

Pneumonias and severe skin and soft tissue infections should be treated aggressively. Despite the frequency of infectious complications, the role of perioperative antibiotics in tracheostomy remains controversial.[2,31]

Cutaneous Fistula

After decannulation, most stomas close in approximately 6 weeks. Persistent epithelialization of the stoma track can result in fistula formation. If the stoma persists after 3 to 6 months, a tracheocutaneous fistula is diagnosed.[3] Persistent tracheocutaneous fistulas can lead to skin irritation and infection due to draining secretions, weak cough, and aspiration leading to recurrent pneumonias, poor phonation, poor cosmesis, and submersion intolerance.[33] The most notable risk factor is prolonged tracheostomy tube placement with one small series noting tracheostomy placement for at least a year in all observed cases.[2] Other risk factors include steroid use, advanced age, and malnutrition.[3] Management options include tract cauterization or excision with healing by secondary intention or surgical closure.[3,33]

SUMMARY

With more than 110,000 tracheostomies being placed annually in the United States, the emergency provider must be prepared to deal with both catastrophic and urgent tracheostomy-related emergencies. Life-threatening complications, including accidental decannulation, obstruction, and hemorrhage, are rare but require immediate action. Having a predetermined, stepwise approach to these complications will help guide management when such patients arrive in the ED.

Subacute complications, such as tracheoesophageal fistula formation, tracheal stenosis, infection, and cutaneous fistula formation, may occur at any time, ranging from the postoperative period to years after a tracheostomy was placed or even following decannulation.

The emergency provider must maintain a high index of suspicion for a tracheostomy-related complication when a patient with a present or prior tracheostomy presents with fever, dyspnea, or hemoptysis.

REFERENCES

1. Shah RK, Lander L, Berry JG, et al. Tracheotomy outcomes and complications: a national perspective. Laryngoscope 2012;122(1):25–9.
2. Goldenberg D, Ari EG, Golz A, et al. Tracheotomy complications: a retrospective study of 1130 cases. Otolaryngol Head Neck Surg 2000;123(3):495–500.
3. Fernandez-Bussy S, Mahajan B, Folch E, et al. Tracheostomy tube placement: early and late complications. J Bronchology Interv Pulmonol 2015;22(4):357–64.
4. Cheung NH, Napolitano LM. Tracheostomy: epidemiology, indications, timing, technique, and outcomes. Respir Care 2014;59(6):895–919.
5. Weiss AJ, Elixhauser A, Steiner C. Readmission to US hospitals by procedure, 2010: statistical brief #154. Healthcare cost and utilization Project (HCUP)

statistical briefs. Rockville (MD): Agency for Healthcare Research and Quality (US); 2006–2013. p. 1–17.

6. Das P, Zhu H, Shah RK, et al. Tracheotomy-related catastrophic events: results of a national survey. Laryngoscope 2012;122(1):30–7.

7. McWhorter AJ. Tracheotomy: timing and techniques. Curr Opin Otolaryngol Head Neck Surg 2003;11(6):473–9.

8. Oliver ER, Gist A, Gillespie MB. Percutaneous versus surgical tracheotomy: an updated meta-analysis. Laryngoscope 2007;117:1570–5.

9. Heffner JE, Miller S, Sahn SA. Tracheostomy in the intensive care unit: part 1: indications, technique, management. Chest 1986;90:269–74.

10. Yaghoobi S, Kayalha H, Ghafouri R, et al. Comparison of complications in percutaneous dilatational tracheostomy versus surgical tracheostomy. Glob J Health Sci 2014;6(4):221–5.

11. Cipriano A, Mao ML, Hon HH, et al. An overview of complications associated with open and percutaneous tracheostomy procedures. Int J Crit Illn Inj Sci 2015;5(3): 179–88.

12. Kapadia FN, Tekawade PC, Nath SS, et al. A prolonged observational study of tracheal tube displacements: benchmarking an incidence <0.5-1% in a medical-surgical adult intensive care unit. Indian J Crit Care Med 2014;18(5): 273–7.

13. Friedman Y, Fildes J, Mizock B, et al. Comparison of percutaneous and surgical tracheostomies. Chest 1996;110(2):480–5.

14. Kremer B, Botos-Kremer AI, Eckel HE, et al. Indications, complications, and surgical techniques for pediatric tracheostomies–an update. J Pediatr Surg 2002; 37(11):1556–62.

15. McGrath B, Bates L, Atkinson D, et al, National Tracheostomy Safety Project. Multidisciplinary guidelines for the management of tracheostomy and laryngectomy airway emergencies. Anaesthesia 2012;67(9):1025–41.

16. Lerner AD, Yarmus L. Percutaneous dilational tracheostomy. Clin Chest Med 2018;39:211–2.

17. O'Connor HH, White AC. Tracheostomy decannulation. Respir Care 2010;55(8): 1076–81.

18. Mitchell RB, Hussey HM, Setzen G, et al. Clinical consensus statement: tracheostomy care. Otolaryngol Head Neck Surg 2013;148(1):6–20.

19. Lyons MJ, Cooke J, Cochrane LA, et al. Safe reliable atraumatic replacement of misplaced paediatric tracheostomy tubes. Int J Pediatr Otorhinolaryngol 2007; 71(11):1743–6.

20. Klancir T, Adam VN, Mršić V, et al. Bilateral pneumothorax as a complication of percutaneous tracheostomy: case report. Acta Clin Croat 2016;55(Suppl 1): 98–102.

21. Bradley PJ. Bleeding around a tracheostomy wound: what to consider and what to do? J Laryngol Otol 2009;123(9):952–6.

22. Scalise P, Prunk SR, Healy D, et al. The incidence of tracheoarterial fistula in patients with chronic tracheostomy tubes: a retrospective study of 544 patients in a long-term care facility. Chest 2005;128(6):3906–9.

23. Wang RC, Perlman PW, Parnes SM. Near-fatal complications of tracheotomy infections and their prevention. Head Neck 1989;11(6):528–33.

24. Reger B, Neu R, Hofmann HS, et al. High mortality in patients with tracheoarterial fistulas: clinical experience and treatment recommendations. Interact Cardiovasc Thorac Surg 2018;26(1):12–7.

25. Jones JW, Reynolds M, Hewitt RL, et al. Tracheo-innominate artery erosion: successful surgical management of a devastating complication. Ann Surg 1976; 184(2):194–204.

26. Allan JS, Wright CD. Tracheoinnominate fistula: diagnosis and management. Chest Surg Clin N Am 2003;13:331–41.

27. Paraschiv M. Tracheoesophageal fistula–a complication of prolonged tracheal intubation. J Med Life 2014;7(4):516–21.

28. Menezes RG, Pant S, Prasad SC, et al. An autopsy case of iatrogenic tracheoesophageal fistula secondary to tracheostomy. Am J Forensic Med Pathol 2014; 35(2):77–9.

29. Epstein SK. Late complications of tracheostomy. Respir Care 2005;50:542–9.

30. Zias N, Chroneou A, Tabba MK, et al. Post tracheostomy and post intubation tracheal stenosis: report of 31 cases and review of the literature. BMC Pulm Med 2008;8:18.

31. Sittitrai P, Siriwittayakorn C. Perioperative antibiotic prophylaxis in open tracheostomy: a preliminary randomized controlled trial. Int J Surg 2018;54(Pt A):170–5.

32. Sharif KF, Baik FM, Jategaonkar AA, et al. Septic arthritis of the sternoclavicular joint: a unique late complication after tracheostomy. Am J Otolaryngol 2018. https://doi.org/10.1016/j.amjoto.2018.05.005.

33. Wine TM, Simons JP, Mehta DK. Comparison of 2 techniques of tracheocutaneous fistula closure. JAMA Otolaryngol Head Neck Surg 2014;140(3):237–42.

Foreign Bodies of the Ear, Nose and Throat

Leslie C. Oyama, MD

KEYWORDS

- Ear foreign bodies • Nose foreign bodies • Throat foreign bodies
- ENT Foreign bodies

KEY POINTS

- Adult and pediatric patients who present to the emergency department with a variety of chief complaints may ultimately be found to have ear, nose, or throat foreign bodies.
- Removal of these foreign bodies requires knowledge and skill.
- For the majority of foreign bodies encountered, it is within the scope of practice of an emergency department practitioner to attempt removal, however, specialty consultation may be needed in some cases.
- In the case of foreign bodies to the nose and throat, particular care must be taken with regards to airway protection.

INTRODUCTION

Ear, nose, and throat foreign bodies may be encountered in outpatient clinics and emergency department (ED) visits. Both adult and pediatric patients may present with this chief complaint. The etiology of these foreign bodies may or may not be known. Particularly in those cases when the etiology is unknown, the presenting complaint may be pain or discomfort, and without a history that points to the diagnosis of foreign body, the diagnosis may be missed. Avoiding premature closure and performing a thorough physical examination will aid in the process of discovering a foreign body as the etiology of a patient's complaint. Foreign bodies of the ear and nose often can be managed in the outpatient setting without significant risk. Foreign bodies in the throat are often medical emergencies that could potentially progress to surgical emergencies. Care must be maintained while examining for a potential foreign body in the throat so as not to cause an acute airway complication. Imaging may or may not aid in diagnosis of a foreign body to the ear, nose, or throat. Both an understanding of the anatomy involved as well as an understanding of the most appropriate setting for removal are important to the successful and safe removal of

Department of Emergency Medicine, UC San Diego, 200 West Arbor Drive, MC 8676, San Diego, CA 92103-8676, USA
E-mail address: loyama@ucsd.edu

Emerg Med Clin N Am 37 (2019) 121–130
https://doi.org/10.1016/j.emc.2018.09.009   emed.theclinics.com
0733-8627/19/© 2018 Elsevier Inc. All rights reserved.

these foreign bodies with the goal of avoiding progression to an acute clinical deterioration. Although there are no gold standard methodologies for foreign body removal, several common removal techniques are reviewed. Removal techniques often use topical anesthesia, irrigation, suction, and/or forceps.

Considerations for successful removal of foreign bodies in the ear, nose, and throat are multifactorial, including patient compliance with removal, which may be limited by age, mental status, pain, compliance with examination/removal, shape of object, density of foreign body, visibility of object, size of object and dexterity and experience of the treating provider.

Foreign Bodies: Ear

Ear canal foreign bodies can present in a wide variety of ways. They can be asymptomatic or may manifest as ear pain, infection, purulent drainage from affected ear, decreased hearing, hyperacusis, itching, or the sensation of foreign body in the ear. Most adults with normal mental status know the etiology of the foreign body. Young pediatric patients and patients with altered mental status often do not know the etiology of the foreign body to the ear. Considerations of what the foreign body of unknown etiology might be may be elicited by history (ie, retained cotton swab after use or live insect, particularly if given a history of the sensation of movement from within the ear).

Examination of the ear and removal of the foreign body from the external auditory canal may provoke pain. The anatomy of the inner ear consists of an external segment that is surrounded by cartilage and then bony canal covered by periosteum. Both are covered by a thin layer of skin. The canal itself usually has 2 areas that are anatomically narrow. The duration of time that the foreign body has been in the ear may contribute to inflammation, ulceration, and bleeding before any attempt at foreign body removal. Because this is true, it is important to try to minimize serial examinations and attempts at removing the foreign body. An otoscope and a strong light source should be used to identify the foreign body before any attempts at removal occur. Topical anesthesia also may be of utility to assist in the extrication. Laboratory tests are not indicated and advanced imaging is usually not needed. Computed tomography (CT) may be helpful if infection or erosion is suspected, particularly if the foreign body has been present for a prolonged period.

Risks associated with removal of foreign bodies in the ear include bleeding, unintentionally lodging the foreign body deeper in the canal, incomplete removal, or perforation of the tympanic membrane. The most commonly occurring complications in pediatric series are external ear canal bleeding (approximately 16%), otitis externa (6%), and tympanic membrane perforation (2%).[1] Uncommon but potential otologic complications of ear canal foreign body removal include damage to the ossicular chain, sensorineural hearing loss, vertigo, facial nerve paralysis, and meningitis.[2]

In most cases, foreign body removal attempts may occur in the ED. Presence of a foreign body for more than 24 hours or in a very young patient (younger than 4 years) does not constitute an independent risk factor for foreign body removal failure or complication. The emergency physician may thus proceed with removal efforts if not otherwise contraindicated.[3] Successful removal of the foreign body can be facilitated by minimizing attempts at removal, pain management, suitable visualization of foreign body, proper equipment, dexterity, and a cooperative patient.

Pain management

Consider topical anesthesia with warm nonviscous lidocaine 1% to aid in anesthesia of the affected ear and management of pain. Other options include 2% lidocaine, alcohol, or mineral oil. Viscous lidocaine may make visualization and removal of object more challenging. Instillation of medications or solutions at cold temperatures may trigger a caloric response. Other options for pain management include injecting lidocaine 1% within the auditory canal with a tuberculin needle at 4 quadrants of the canal (12, 3, 6, and 9 o'clock) using the otoscope, procedural sedation, or general anesthesia. Available data suggest that approximately 95% of aural foreign bodies can be removed without the need for general anesthesia.[4]

Adequate visualization

The ear canal has 2 areas where it narrows: one at the cartilaginous portion of the canal and one at the bony portion of the inner ear. On examination, a gentle posterior and superior pull of the pinna will help optimize the view of the ear canal along with immobilization of the head. A strong light source that can be found on a head lamp and a large-size speculum on an otoscope will be of high utility in the aid of visualizing within the canal.

Equipment

Consider having the following equipment available before beginning the procedure (**Fig. 1**):

1. Frazier suction
2. Alligator forceps
3. Cerumen loop

Foreign body composition and approach to removal

Consideration of the material comprising the foreign body to be removed is important in facilitating successful removal.

Solid, noncompressible foreign body removal Examples of solid, noncompressible foreign bodies to the ear include hair beads, toys, button batteries, food products, and rocks.

- Removal by forceps:
  - If the object is known to be a solid, noncompressible object, forceps that can grasp the diameter of the object should be selected. If the available forceps can neither be inserted along the periphery of the object between the object and the external auditory canal nor grasp the diameter of the object, another approach may be more successful.

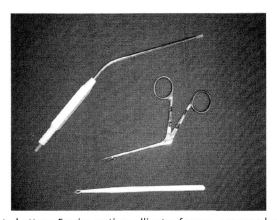

Fig. 1. From top to bottom: Frazier suction, alligator forceps, cerumen loop.

- Removal by cerumen loop:
  - If the solid noncompressible object is small enough, it may be possible to use a cerumen loop passed between the object and the wall of the eustachian canal. Use the slightly angled part of the instrument to get behind the object and pull the object out of the ear.
  - This technique may be particularly useful with smooth or solid objects that are slick or slippery.
- Removal by Frazier suction:
  - A Frazier suction can be connected to continuous low suction and applied directly on to the object. Occlude the insufflation port to suction out the contents of the patient's ear canal. Of note, the strength of the suction may not be enough to remove the object.
- Removal by sterile swab stick with medical glue adhesive:
  - This technique includes use of a sterile swab: specifically the end of the swab without the cotton or rayon tip. Use the other end of the swab and place a very small amount of medical adhesive glue on the tip. This technique may be particularly useful in the removal of a round object that may be hard to grasp with forceps. The medical adhesive glue on the back end of the stick of the swab may then be carefully and gently placed directly on the object. Use great care not to advance the foreign body farther into the eustachian canal or misdirect the glued end inadvertently to the eustachian canal itself. After holding the glued end of the swab stick against the solid object for a few seconds, the adhesive will have dried, which will allow manual removal of the foreign body at the end of the glued stick and these will now be removed as one unit.

Compressible foreign body removal Examples of compressible foreign bodies to the ear include retained tips of cotton swabs or pieces of paper that have been used in attempts at cleaning the ear canal.

- Removal by suction:
  - A Frazier suction can be connected to continuous low suction and applied directly onto the object. Occlude the insufflation port to suction out the contents of the patient's ear canal. Of note, the strength of the suction may not be enough to remove the object. Suction may avoid creating additional debris by inadvertent destruction of the object during the removal process. Creating debris should be avoided.[4]
- Removal by water irrigation:
  - Items needed:
    - Warm water (to avoid caloric response)
    - Basin (to catch irrigated water)
    - 60-mL syringe
    - Angiocath (intravenous needle removed)
  - Fill the syringe with warm water
  - Attach the plastic angiocath to the syringe
  - Insert the angiocath next to or behind the foreign body (if possible)
  - Irrigate the ear by emptying the syringe through the angiocath
  - Observe for the foreign body to become dislodged. It will subsequently exit the canal with irrigation
  - Avoid this technique with objects that might expand (ie, food products) or button batteries (to avoid battery current that may induce liquefaction necrosis)

Special considerations

- Insects:
  - History:
    - When a patient complains of "movement" or "fluttering" inside the ear along with foreign body sensation, the presence of an insect should be considered.[5] Additionally, a history of recent camping activity or poor living conditions may prompt a concern for an insect within the ear canal. In most cases, the insect is a cockroach.[6]
  - Examination:
    - Light-avoiding insects (such as cockroaches) will often be stimulated to move when an examiner's light is used to examine the ear. This may cause discomfort or provoke anxiety to the patient.
  - Removal of an insect from the ear:
    - First, anesthetize and euthanize the insect. Various success rates have been reported with various used agents. Efficacious formulations include lidocaine as a 10% spray or less concentrated liquid, 2% lidocaine gel, mineral oil with 2% or 4% lidocaine, and alcohol. One study suggested that microscope immersion oil is more efficacious than lidocaine preparations.[5] Given the viscosity of oil and gel, nonviscous agents will aid in maintaining a good visual field for removal of the insect.
    - Instill nonviscous lidocaine into the ear and wait several minutes. Once inactivity is noted, proceed on to extraction. The Frazier suction may most efficiently extract the insect intact and will avoid creating debris that can be caused by manual extraction.[7]
- Styrofoam may be dissolved with acetone.
- Cyanoacrylate glue may be loosened/dissolved with acetone.
- When not to attempt foreign body removal:
  - The foreign body is sharp and likely to cause more trauma on an attempt to remove
  - Evidence of perforated tympanic membrane on initial inspection
- When to call consultant (otolaryngology):
  - Unable to remove foreign body (especially if button battery, as these will erode the ear canal).
  - Immunocompromised patient with evidence of infection. Needs close outpatient follow-up at minimum.

Foreign Bodies: Nose

Foreign bodies to the nose are most commonly seen in children, mentally challenged, and psychiatric patients. Although they may be located anywhere within the nasal cavity, they are most commonly located in or around the floor of the nose just below the inferior turbinate or immediately anterior to the middle turbinate.[8] If a history is unable to be obtained, one must pay careful attention to signs and symptoms exhibited by the patient, which may include unilateral nare obstruction, pain, nasal discharge, epistaxis, sinus pain, or possibly aspiration of the foreign body if it dislodged posteriorly from the nose and traveled down the airway. Without maintaining a high index of suspicion, a misdiagnosis may occur that could result in sinusitis, inflammation, or encrustation of the object within the sinus. The list of objects that have been reportedly removed from the nose is extensive and limited seemingly only by the size of the nostril. It is suggested that because most people are right-handed, most nasal foreign bodies are right-sided.[9]

Foreign body composition

Consideration of the material comprising the foreign body to be removed will be useful in successfully removing the foreign body. Objects are usually inanimate or animate. The most commonly identified inanimate foreign bodies include rubber erasers, paper wads, pebbles, beads, marbles, beans, safety pins, washers, nuts, sponges, and chalk.[8] Myiasis of the nose is common in warm tropical climates of the southwestern United States and the Far East, including India. The frequency of infestation is primarily related to the poor hygiene of the inhabitants due to their living conditions.[10] The most common of all infestations is the fly maggot. Screwworms, also known as "Texas" screwworms are serious pests to humans and cattle.[10]

Diagnostics

If the foreign body is visualized on physical examination, imaging may not be necessary. If, however, the patient is unable to provide a history or placement of the object was unwitnessed, imaging with a plain film of the sinus may be considered. If there is any suspicion for a button battery as the possible etiology of the object, plain radiographs may be of great utility and a low-threshold to use plain radiography should be maintained when button-battery foreign bodies are suspected.[11] If the foreign body is unable to be directly visualized, CT scan may be helpful. Caution is advised in consideration of using MRI if there is any concern that the foreign body may have a magnetic component.[12] Be advised that many facial body piercings use magnets, making this etiology of foreign body even more worrisome for necrosis if tissue is caught between the magnets or if MRI is used.

Approach to removal

There are several different approaches that can be used to remove a nasal foreign body. Before attempting removal, the patient may benefit from some combination of restraint, sedation, and pretreatment with vasoconstrictive agents (eg, nebulized racemic epinephrine) and anesthetic (eg, benzocaine spray).[13] Approaches to removal include positive pressure techniques, suction, instruments, magnets, and/or medical adhesive glue.

Positive pressure technique A quick burst of air into the mouth of the patient with the unaffected nare occluded may result in spontaneous removal of the object. The burst of air may be delivered by

- A bag valve mask with the unaffected nare occluded
- Having a breath delivered by a parent to their child as if they were going to give them a kiss with the unaffected nare occluded
- The patient taking a deep breath then blowing out through the nose with the unaffected nare occluded

The "kiss" technique's success rate of nearly 50% was associated with additional advantages of decreased use of resources (eg, time, anesthetics).[14]

Removal by suction This technique may be used successfully if the object appears to be loose within the nasal cavity or if organic matter is suspected (to avoid further degradation of the material on removal). Use of a Frazier suction catheter to low wall suction may successfully remove these types of foreign bodies.

Removal with instruments
- Alligator forceps may be used in removing solid, nonorganic, inanimate objects. Alligator forceps can be used to grab the object directly.

- A right-angle blunt-tipped probe may be used in removing solid, nonorganic, inanimate objects. A right-angle blunt-tipped probe may be able to go around the object and pull it out from the object's posterior side.
- A pediatric Foley (5F or 6F) can be used in the same manner by placing sterile lubricant or viscous lidocaine to the distal end of the Foley and inserting it past the object. If this is achieved, insufflate the Foley balloon once it is to the posterior side of the object and then gently pull the Foley anteriorly, thus pulling the object out of the nose.
- Snare technique: This technique is used to help dislodge an object that may be wedged in the turbinate, making removal challenging. A 24-gauge wire "snare" loop can be created using a 10-cm section with both ends in a clamp. This snare can then be inserted into the nasal aperture and used to dissect a plane between the object and the septum, turbinate, and nasal floor mucosa to free all sides of the object.[15] Use of oxymetazoline (0.05%) nasal spray and a lidocaine with epinephrine before this will aid in vasoconstriction of the mucosa and help minimize bleeding.

Removal with magnet This technique can be used for suspected metallic foreign bodies.

Removal with medical adhesive glue Cyanoacrylate tissue glue may be applied to the handle of a cotton swab then directly applied to a clearly visualized object and held in place for approximately 60 seconds. This will allow time for the glue to adhere to the object and the foreign body can then be pulled out as the handle of the swab will have affixed itself to the object. Great care must be used so as not to have the glue contact healthy tissue instead of the foreign body.

Risks and complications
Risks for foreign body removal from the nose include bleeding, infection, and dislodgement into the airway. Sedation is discouraged because it can increase complications by reducing the gag and cough reflexes.[16] Foreign objects that have been forcefully inserted, have become encrusted due to prolonged retention in the nasal cavity, or live and mobile animate foreign bodies (ie, maggots, larvae) pose increased difficulty in removal.[10]

Consultation should be obtained when the foreign body cannot be removed or adequately visualized, or when a tumor or mass is suspected.[17]

Foreign Bodies: Throat

Foreign bodies to the throat can be approached in various ways depending on various factors. Things to consider: (1) Is the patient is stable or unstable? (2) What is the anatomic location of the object (proximal or distal airway)? (3) What are the possible etiologies of the foreign body (based on age pediatric or elderly)?

Airway: stable or unstable
Foreign bodies to the throat may present acutely with respiratory distress. The fact that the incidence peaks in the very young and very old may help explain delays in diagnosis for subacute cases, as specific and reliable indicators of airway foreign body presence are often elusive.[18] Patients with foreign bodies to the throat may present acutely with the need for immediate airway stabilization. Those patients who are stable likely have a partial airway obstruction and great care must be taken to avoid converting a patent airway to a complete obstruction with diagnostic or therapeutic maneuvers.

Anatomy

Adult anatomy results in predilection for foreign bodies to be located in the proximal airways (larynx, trachea, main bronchi). In children, fewer than half of foreign objects are located proximally and instead are more commonly located in within the bronchial tree.[19]

Population and etiologies

Foreign bodies in the airway are commonly seen in the pediatric population.[17,19] One case series over a 20-year period reported that 75% of patients with foreign bodies to the airway were younger than 9 years.[19] Peak incidence of aspiration is in the second year of life, with a dramatic decline after age 3.[20] The peak incidence of aspiration in adults occurs in the elderly population.[21] Materials that are noted prevalently as foreign bodies to the throat include fractured, broken, avulsed teeth; a dental apparatus; or items intended for the gastrointestinal system: primarily meats and medications.[22] Other common foreign bodies are items that were temporarily placed and held in the patient's mouth, such as pins, needles, jewelry, or thermometers. Also included are items being explored by young toddlers, such as small toys. In the pediatric population, almost half of fatal choking cases were a result of food aspiration, with hot dogs (17%), candy (10%), nuts (9%), and grapes (8%) most frequently reported.[23]

Because pediatric foreign bodies to the airway are usually located in the bronchial tree, bronchial obstruction is of great concern and may lead to hypoxemia. Incomplete bronchial obstructions may present on examination as a wheeze, unequal breath sounds, cough, stridor, or potentially no obvious findings on clinical examination. Although adults often have foreign bodies lodge in the right main stem bronchus (69% of bronchial foreign bodies were right-sided),[24] the pediatric population has shown a more equal left-right distribution of lower airway foreign bodies.[21]

Diagnostics

In the stable patient, plain radiography of the neck and chest remain the mainstay of airway foreign body imaging.[24] In children with airway foreign bodies, chest radiograph findings are frequently normal and can display abnormalities uncharacteristic for foreign body aspiration. Inspiratory and expiratory films may reveal air trapping, but bronchoscopy and micro laryngoscopy (with an operating microscope) remain the ultimate diagnostic modalities.[20,25] Children witnessed to choke while having small particles in their mouth who subsequently are noted to have raspy respiration, wheezing, or coughing, should undergo prompt bronchoscopy regardless of radiographic findings.[25]

Treatment

Treatment of foreign bodies to the throat usually involves removal. If the patient is stable, and the foreign body is proximal to the oropharynx, the ED physician may attempt removal. Direct laryngoscopic visualization during intubation may reveal a proximal foreign object that can be removed with Magill forceps.[22] Foreign bodies that are not removed may later result in infection or perforation. Early bronchoscopy in any patient with a suspected foreign body is key to reducing morbidity and mortality, and the role of endoscopic management remains important given limitations of other diagnostic methods.[20] Patients who are unstable due to a critical airway obstruction require immediate airway stabilization. If there is no air movement, the patient is unable to phonate, and if the patient appears hypoxic, the patient may be choking and the Heimlich maneuver could be considered. This is not usually encountered in the ED setting, as the patient will likely lose consciousness shortly after an upper airway complete obstruction occurs. Treatment of foreign bodies in the upper airway in the

ED may first be accomplished with orotracheal intubation. If there is a complete obstruction of the oropharynx, cricothyrotomy may be the best airway management option. If the obstructing foreign body is more distal, pushing the object farther down into the distal bronchus is a consideration if it is unable to removed. Another strategy in this situation could be to use a pharyngeotracheal lumen airway, which is a double-lumen endotracheal tube that is inserted blindly into the pharynx. After the position of the tube has been assessed, the patient is ventilated through the appropriate lumen. A large pharyngeal balloon seals the airway and a smaller secondary balloon is then inflated. The published complication rate is low, but there has been relatively little evaluation of this device.[25–28]

SUMMARY

Foreign bodies to the ear, nose, and throat often can be managed in the ED, particularly if the patient offers a history consistent with foreign body and is calm and compliant with the examination and removal attempts. Tips for success include analgesia, adequate visualization, immobilization of the patient's head, dexterity and experience level of the provider, and minimizing attempts at removal. It is critical to recognize the risks involved with certain retained objects (button batteries or sharp objects), as well as when to call a consultant to help facilitate safe, successful removal of objects to the ear, nose, and throat.

REFERENCES

1. Marin JR, Trainor JL. Foreign body removal from the external auditory canal in a pediatric emergency department. Pediatr Emerg Care 2006;22(9):630–4.
2. Dance D, Riley M, Ludemann P. Removal of ear canal foreign bodies in children: what can go wrong and when to refer. BC Medical Journal 2009;51:20–4.
3. Ologe FE, Dunmade AD, Afolabi OA. Aural foreign bodies in children. Indian J Pediatr 2007;74(8):755–8.
4. Tintinalli JE, Stapczynski SJ. Tintinalli's emergency medicine: a comprehensive study guide. 7th edition. New York: McGraw-Hill; 2011. p. 1556.
5. Bhargava D, Victor R. Carabid beetle invasion of the ear in Oman. Wilderness Environ Med 1999;10(3):157–60.
6. Indudharan R, Ahamad M, Ho TM, et al. Human otoacariasis. Ann Trop Med Parasitol 1999;93(2):163–7.
7. Leffler S, Cheney P, Tandberg D. Chemical immobilization and killing of intra-aural roaches: an in vitro comparative study. Ann Emerg Med 1993;22(12):1795–8.
8. DeWeese D, Saunders AH. Acute and chronic diseases of the nose. In: DeWeese DD, Saunders AH, editors. Textbook of otolaryngology. St Louis (MO): CV Mosby; 1982.
9. Okoye BC, Onotai LO. Foreign bodies in the nose. Niger J Med 2006;15(3): 301–4.
10. Kalan A, Tariq M. Foreign bodies in the nasal cavities: a comprehensive review of the aetiology, diagnostic pointers, and therapeutic measures. Postgrad Med J 2000;76(898):484–7.
11. Glynn F, Amin M, Kinsella J. Nasal foreign bodies in children: Should they have a plain radiograph in the accident and emergency? Pediatr Emerg Care 2008; 24(4):217–8.
12. Yeh B, Roberson JR. Nasal magnetic foreign body: a sticky topic. J Emerg Med 2012;43(2):319–21.

13. Douglas AR. Use of nebulized adrenaline to aid expulsion of intra-nasal foreign bodies in children. J Laryngol Otol 1996;110(6):559–60.
14. Taylor C, Acheson J, Coats TJ. Nasal foreign bodies in children: kissing it better. Emerg Med J 2010;27(9):712–3.
15. Fundakowski CE, Moon S, Torres L. The snare technique: a novel atraumatic method for the removal of difficult nasal foreign bodies. J Emerg Med 2013; 44(1):104–6.
16. Kadish H. Ear and nose foreign bodies: "It is all about the tools." Clin Pediatr (Phila) 2005;44(8):665–70.
17. Heim SW, Maughan KL. Foreign bodies in the ear, nose, and throat. Am Fam Physician 2007;76(8):1185–9.
18. Higuchi O, Adachi Y, Ichimaru T, et al. Foreign body aspiration in children: a nationwide survey in Japan. Int J Pediatr Otorhinolaryngol 2009;73(5):659–61.
19. Baharloo F, Veyckemans F, Francis C, et al. Tracheobronchial foreign bodies: presentation and management in children and adults. Chest 1999;115(5):1357–62.
20. Righini CA, Morel N, Karkas A, et al. What is the diagnostic value of flexible bronchoscopy in the initial investigation of children with suspected foreign body aspiration? Int J Pediatr Otorhinolaryngol 2007;71(9):1383–90.
21. Bodart E, de Bilderling G, Tuerlinckx D, et al. Foreign body aspiration in childhood: management algorithm. Eur J Emerg Med 1989;6(1):21–5.
22. Soroudi A, Shipp HE, Stepanski BM, et al. Adult foreign body airway obstruction in the prehospital setting. Prehosp Emerg Care 2007;11(1):25–9.
23. Harris CS, Baker SP, Smith GA, et al. Childhood asphyxiation by food. A national analysis and overview. JAMA 1984;251(17):2231–5.
24. Kavanagh PV, Mason AC, Muller NL. Thoracic foreign bodies in adults. Clin Radiol 1999;54(6):353–60.
25. Zerella J, Dimler A, McGill L, et al. Foreign body aspiration in children: value of radiography and complications of bronchoscopy. J Pediatr Surg 1998;33(11): 1651–4.
26. AARC (American Association for Respiratory Care) clinical practice guideline. Management of airway emergencies. Respir Care 1995;40(7):749–60.
27. Niemann JT, Rosborough JP, Myers R, et al. The pharyngeo-tracheal lumen airway: preliminary investigations of a new adjunct. Ann Emerg Med 1984; 13(8):591–6.
28. Bartlett RL, Martin SD, McMahon JM, et al. A field comparison of the pharyngeotracheal lumen airway and the endotracheal tube. J Trauma 1992;32(3):280–4.

Traumatic Injuries of the Ear, Nose and Throat

Mac Henry, MD[a], H. Gene Hern, MD[b],*

KEYWORDS

- Facial injuries • Airway • Tracheal injury • Hematoma • Nasal septum
- Tympanic membrane

KEY POINTS

- Airway injuries must be considered in patients with dyspnea, tachypnea, voice changes, abnormal respirations, or poor oxygen saturation.
- After an auricular hematoma is drained, the skin should be closed and sutured to the underlying cartilage to prevent reaccumulation.
- The possibility of domestic violence and nonaccidental trauma should always be assessed when interviewing patients with nasal trauma.
- Most traumatic tympanic membrane ruptures will heal with time and do not require emergent intervention.

INTRODUCTION

Soft tissue trauma of the head and neck presents a variety of considerations for the emergency physician, including complex airway management and wound repair. Physical examination of any trauma patient should be complete and include careful airway evaluation and management. Special attention should be given to injuries such as septal and auricular hematomas where prompt, appropriate wound care can prevent significant long-term sequelae. This article highlights 4 areas of special importance: airway trauma, septal and auricular hematoma, and tympanic membrane rupture.

AIRWAY TRAUMA

Airway trauma is a rare manifestation of head and neck trauma. Often accompanied by other injuries, the emergency physician must maintain a high index of suspicion for

Disclosure Statement: The authors do not have any disclosures.
[a] Alameda Health System, Highland Hospital, 1411 East 31st, Oakland, CA 94602, USA;
[b] Emergency Medicine, Alameda Health System, Highland Hospital, 1411 East 31st, Oakland, CA 94602, USA
* Corresponding author.
E-mail address: emergentt@gmail.com

acute airway injury when assessing trauma patients, and consider alternatives to rapid-sequence intubation when intubation is required for these patients.

The true incidence of laryngeal trauma is unknown. Estimates range from 1:5000 to 1:137,000 trauma patients.[1–4] Among trauma patients with penetrating neck injuries, the incidence of laryngeal injury is 15%.[1] Death from airway injuries before emergency department (ED) presentation has been estimated to be as high as 80%.[1,5] In-hospital mortality ranges from 2% to 15%.[1,2] As many as 50% of patients with laryngeal trauma will have other injuries,[1] so a careful airway examination and a high index of suspicion must be maintained when evaluating any trauma patient.

Laryngeal trauma can result from blunt or penetrating injury. Blunt injury may be from motor vehicle accidents involving rapid deceleration and compression of the neck between the cervical spine and an airbag, dashboard, or seatbelt; so-called clothesline injuries of riders of motorcycles or all-terrain vehicles when struck to the neck by a fixed object; or by strangulation or hanging.[1] Blunt trauma to the superior thorax can also cause laryngeal injury if there is a forceful expulsion of air against a closed glottis.[3] Penetrating injuries are typically caused by shooting or stabbing.

Evaluation of a patient with an acute presentation and suspected airway injury should include advanced traumatic life support primary and secondary surveys. Spinal precautions should be observed and cervical spine injury assumed. The examiner will likely need assistance in removing a cervical collar and having an assistant hold the cervical spine in line while the examiner makes a close inspection of the neck. Penetrating trauma is more likely to be obvious than blunt trauma, but either can be overlooked, particularly in a patient with polytrauma.[2] The emergency physician should make a careful assessment of the airway, including inspection for midline trachea, cervical bruising or penetration injuries, and palpation for subcutaneous emphysema. Airway injuries must be considered in patients with dyspnea, tachypnea, voice changes, abnormal respirations, or poor oxygen saturation.[2–4]

Delayed presentation of these injuries is also possible. Patients with blunt trauma to the neck may initially have a stable airway but may develop swelling and airway compromise subsequently.[4] All patients with trauma to the neck should be observed in a high-visibility area.[4] Laryngeal trauma also should be kept in the differential when evaluating patients with hoarseness, voice changes, anterior neck discomfort, or bruising. A history of recent endoscopy or intubation should be elicited, and iatrogenic airway trauma considered.[5]

Special consideration should be given to advanced airway management in patients with confirmed or suspected airway injury. Rapid-sequence intubation may be dangerous in these patients for several reasons. Patients with laryngeal trauma may be maintaining their airway only through muscle tone, and paralysis can cause airway collapse. Further, direct laryngoscopy, even with a video laryngoscope, does not allow airway visualization past the vocal cords. Blind placement of an endotracheal tube below the cords may result in the creation of a false passage or allow the endotracheal tube to leave the airway altogether through a nonvisualized defect.[4–7] Therefore, awake fiberoptic intubation of patients with laryngeal injuries is preferred. This allows direct visualization of the airway past the vocal cords and prevents the possible creation of a false passage. If time and resources allow, intubation of these patients in the operating room may be preferred.[4] Some sources suggest preparation for surgical airway before beginning intubation, although the effectiveness of cricothyroidotomy in these patients will depend on the location of their injury.[4]

Computerized tomography (CT) scan is the modality of choice in patients with suspected laryngeal injury.[1,4] It can establish the type and extent of injury to the cartilaginous structures of the neck and identify soft tissue injury. Cervical spine CT scans do not typically image far enough anteriorly to be sufficient in suspected airway trauma.[1] There is no consensus guideline for the use of intravenous (IV) contrast, and protocols will vary between institutions. If the airway must be secured emergently, this should happen before the patient is sent to the CT scanner.

Beyond securing the airway, ED management of these patients will depend on the severity of their airway injury, their accompanying injuries, and the resources available to the clinician. Full evaluation of potential airway injuries will require formal endoscopy and often bronchoscopy.[2–5,7] Patients should be admitted for observation to a monitored bed with a low threshold for intensive care unit admission.

Pharmacologic management includes IV steroids. One source recommends either 8 to 10 mg dexamethasone every 8 hours or 250 mg methylprednisolone every 4 hours, starting at the time of presentation and continuing for 24 hours. IV antibiotics can be administered prophylactically or if there are known mucosal injuries. Proton pump inhibitors are also recommended.[2]

AURICULAR AND SEPTAL HEMATOMAS

The close association of skin and cartilage in the external ear and nasal septum creates a risk for long-term sequelae following injury to these tissues. The emergency physician assessing patients with head and neck trauma should pay special attention to the evaluation and emergent management of such wounds to prevent disfiguring scarring.

Auricular Hematoma

An auricular hematoma is a collection of blood between the skin and cartilage of the external ear. It is most common among people playing contact sports, including wrestling, rugby, and mixed martial arts. An auricular hematoma may also suggest nonaccidental trauma or domestic violence. History and physical examination should address this possibility. The injury is caused by shearing forces separating the skin and underlying cartilage and can lead to disfiguring fibrocartilaginous overgrowth, commonly known as cauliflower ear, if the hematoma is not promptly evacuated.[8]

Auricular hematomas typically present with pain out of proportion to the injury, loss of anatomic landmarks on the ear, and a fluctuant mass on the auricle. Patients may present at the time of injury or several days later. The time of injury should be firmly established, as it will determine the best emergency management of the injury as well as the likelihood of favorable cosmetic outcome.[8] The physical examination will help guide treatment, because coagulated hematomas may require more extensive debridement and are best repaired by an otolaryngologist.

Auricular hematomas should be drained and prevented from reaccumulating. A drainage incision should be large enough to allow for irrigation of the space to evacuate clots and fresh blood. The incision should be made in the most anatomically advantageous location to minimize aesthetic effects of scarring.[8–10] After evacuation, blood must not reaccumulate or the hematoma will reform.

Many methods have been proposed and practiced for draining auricular hematoma and preventing reaccumulation. A recent Cochrane review found no superior method due to lack of randomized, controlled trials.[11] We prefer the following method. First the hematoma should be drained with an open incision, as aspiration will not achieve adequate removal of the hematoma.[8–10] The incision should be done along an anatomic fold to minimize scarring. Care should be taken to not incise the cartilage. The hematoma should be evacuated completely and irrigated. Closure is then achieved with absorbable mattress sutures through and through the ear, to ensure adherence of the skin to the cartilage and eliminate potential dead space. The wound should be dressed with ample antibiotic ointment, and can otherwise be left open to the air. Patients should receive tetanus prophylaxis. All patients need to have close follow-up with an otolaryngologist.

Nasal Septal Hematoma

The nasal septum is a cartilaginous structure, which, like the auricle, is susceptible to long-term deformity if robbed of adequate blood supply. Accumulation of blood between the septum and overlying tissue can cause destruction of the septal cartilage and a subsequent "saddle nose" deformity. Hematomas also can become infected, creating a nasal septal abscess with risk of extension of infection into the face and brain.[12,13] Therefore, the emergency physician should evaluate any patient with nasal trauma for a septal hematoma and treat it promptly if found.

Patients may present immediately after trauma or presentation may be delayed. The mechanism of such injuries is typically a direct blow to the nose. The possibility of domestic violence and nonaccidental trauma always should be assessed when interviewing patients with nasal trauma. Children are more susceptible to septal hematomas, possibly because they have softer nasal cartilage than adults, and a thorough examination is particularly important in pediatric patients.[12] Any patient with nasal trauma should be evaluated for further head and facial trauma, and the nose examination should include evaluation for cerebrospinal fluid (CSF) rhinorrhea. CSF rhinorrhea should be suspected in a trauma patient with persistent drainage of clear fluid from the nose. Patients may complain of a sense of fullness or difficulty breathing through their nose, or may complain simply of nasal pain.

Evaluation for nasal septal hematomas requires visualization of the nasal septum, which is not always straightforward in a recently traumatized nose. An otoscope or nasal speculum can be used for visualization. Oxymetazoline nasal spray can help with visualization by reducing mucosal swelling and assist in evacuation of clots or mucus to visualize the septum. A hematoma is described as bluish in color and should be fluctuant, unlike a deviated septum, which may appear bluish but will be firm. If available, a nasal speculum with overhead light source or headlamp can provide better visualization.[13,14]

Once a septal hematoma is identified, the nose can be anesthetized in 2 parts. First by placing elongated cotton balls soaked in a combined solution of 4% lidocaine and oxymetazoline in both nares, then, once that has taken effect in approximately 10 minutes, by direct injection of lidocaine with epinephrine into the hematoma. The hematoma should be incised 5 to 10 mm and drained, with a wound specimen sent for culture if there is concern for abscess. After complete evacuation, the nare should be packed, which is most easily achieved with an inflatable nasal tampon.[15]

All patients with packing should be started on oral antibiotics that cover *Staphylococcus aureus*, including methicillin-resistant *S aureus*, according to local susceptibility patterns. Packing should be removed in 3 days and patients should be provided otolaryngology follow-up.

TRAUMATIC TYMPANIC MEMBRANE RUPTURE

Traumatic tympanic membrane (TM) rupture is associated with blunt and penetrating trauma as well as blast injuries; all mechanisms likely to be encountered in an ED setting. Although treatment of such injuries is typically limited, they are an important consideration for the emergency physician. The mechanism of TM rupture includes penetrating trauma (most commonly with cotton swabs), blunt trauma (blows to the head), and blast injury.[16] Patients may present with complaints of pain, hearing loss, tinnitus, or discharge from the ear. In the case of blast injury, the presence or absence of TM rupture is not an accurate indicator of other injuries. Patients with blast-related TM rupture also should be evaluated for lung injury with a chest radiograph.[17]

Treatment of TM rupture includes careful avoidance of any water in the ear and watchful waiting, as most such injuries will heal with time. Risk factors for nonhealing include penetrating trauma, older age, and ear irrigation following rupture.[18] Patients with significant hearing loss associated with their injury may have ossicular damage and should have prompt evaluation by an otolaryngologist. Any patient with blast-related TM rupture should be seen by an otolaryngologist within 3 to 4 days[19] and all patients with TM rupture require otolaryngology follow-up to assess for healing.[18]

REFERENCES

1. Becker M, Leuchter I, Platon A, et al. Imaging of laryngeal trauma. Eur J Radiol 2014;83(1):142–54.
2. Comer BT, Gal TJ. Recognition and management of the spectrum of acute laryngeal trauma. J Emerg Med 2012;43(5):e289–93.
3. Prokakis C, Koletsis EN, Dedeilias P, et al. Airway trauma: a review on epidemiology, mechanisms of injury, diagnosis and treatment. J Cardiothorac Surg 2014;9:117.
4. Schaefer SD. Management of acute blunt and penetrating external laryngeal trauma. Laryngoscope 2014;124:233–44.
5. Abernathy JH, Reeves ST. Airway catastrophes. Curr Opin Anaesthesiol 2010;23: 41–6.
6. Baumgartner FJ, Ayres B, Theuer C. Danger of false intubation after traumatic tracheal transection. Ann Thorac Surg 1997;63:227–8.
7. Bell RB, Verschueren DS, Dierks EJ. Management of laryngeal trauma. Oral Maxillofac Surg Clin North Am 2008;20(3):415–30.
8. Ghanem T, Rasamny JK, Park SS. Rethinking auricular trauma. Laryngoscope 2005;115:1251.
9. Giles WC, Iverson KC, King JD, et al. Incision and drainage followed by mattress suture repair of auricular hematoma. Laryngoscope 2007;117:2097.
10. Roy S, Smith L. A novel technique for treating auricular hematoma in mixed martial artists (ultimate fighters). Am J Otolaryngol 2010;31:21–4.
11. Jones SE, Mahendran S. Interventions for acute auricular haematoma. Cochrane Database Syst Rev 2004;(2):CD004166.
12. Sanyaolu LN, Farmer SE, Cuddihy PJ. Nasal septal haematoma. BMJ 2014;349: g6075.
13. Landis BM, Borner U. Septal hematoma: always think about it! J Pediatr 2013; 163(4):1223.
14. Puricelli MD, Zitsch RP. Septal hematoma following nasal trauma. J Emerg Med 2016;50(1):121–2.
15. Kass J, Ferguson BJ. Treatment of hematoma of the nasal septum. N Engl J Med 2015;372:e28.
16. Sagiv D, Migirov L, Glikson E, et al. Traumatic perforation of the tympanic membrane: a review of 80 cases. J Emerg Med 2018;54(2):186–90.

17. Shea J, Wei G, Donavan C, et al. Medical management at the explosive incident scene. Ann Emerg Med 2017;69(1S):S20–8.
18. Orji FT, Agu CC. Determinants of spontaneous healing in traumatic perforations of the tympanic membrane. Clin Otolaryngol 2008;33:420–6.
19. Shah A, Ayala M, Capra G, et al. Otologic assessment of blast and nonblast injury in returning Middle East-deployed service members. Laryngoscope 2013;124: 272.

The Diagnosis and Management of Facial Bone Fractures

Steve Chukwulebe, MD[a], Christopher Hogrefe, MD[a,b,c,d],*

KEYWORDS

• Facial • Fracture • Le Fort • Mandibular • Nasal • Orbital • Zygomatic

KEY POINTS

- High-velocity injuries to the face can result in both frontal bone fractures and intracranial injuries. These patients may present with altered mental status.
- When patients incur ocular trauma, the clinician should always test visual acuity because this information can significantly affect a patient's disposition.
- Few individuals with nasal fractures will require a surgical reduction.
- Midface fractures are not as well classified as Le Fort injuries, and most occur in combination with other fractures.
- Possess a high index of suspicion for mandibular fractures in patients with trismus, inability to bite down, or a positive tongue blade bite test.

INTRODUCTION

Facial fractures are a common cause of emergency department (ED) visits, accounting for more than 400,000 annual visits in the United States alone.[1] Traumatic injuries to the face may result in various fracture patterns that can occur in isolation or concomitantly with other injuries. It is important for the treating physician to be mindful of the Airway, Breathing, and Circulation (ABCs) of patient stabilization, as these injuries can compromise a patient's airway or be associated with intracranial and cervical spine injuries. Otherwise, the face itself is composed of 14 bones (not including the cranial frontal bone), and its architecture has evolved to contain several thicker horizontal and

Disclosures: The authors have no financial interests to disclose.
a Department of Emergency Medicine, Northwestern Medicine, Northwestern University Feinberg School of Medicine, 259 East Erie, Suite 1300, Chicago, IL 60611, USA; b Department of Medicine, Northwestern Medicine, Northwestern University Feinber School of Medicine, 259 East Erie Street, Suite 1300, Chicago, IL 60611, USA; c Department of Orthopaedic Surgery, Northwestern Medicine, Northwestern University Feinberg School of Medicine, 259 East Erie Street, Suite 1300, Chicago, IL 60611, USA; d Department of Orthopaedic Surgery, 259 East Erie Street, Suite 1300, Chicago, IL 60611, USA
* Corresponding author. 259 East Erie Street, Suite 1300, Chicago, IL 60611.
E-mail address: christopher.hogrefe@northwestern.edu

Emerg Med Clin N Am 37 (2019) 137–151
https://doi.org/10.1016/j.emc.2018.09.012
0733-8627/19/© 2018 Elsevier Inc. All rights reserved.

vertical buttresses with intervening thinner bones and paranasal sinuses (**Fig. 1**). As a result, this design allows the face to crumple and disperse oncoming anterior and inferior forces away from the cranium.[2]

The epidemiology of facial bone fractures not only differs across populations but has continued to change over the past few decades. **Table 1** lists the factors influencing these changes. In the United States, the most common causes of facial fractures in the adult population are assaults and motor vehicle collisions (MVCs).[3] Other mechanisms, such as falls, sports injuries (commonly head-to-head collision or an elbow to the face), occupational accidents, and gunshot wounds comprise a smaller percentage.[3,4] Although the frequency of the involved bones in facial fractures varies, the underlying mechanism may predict the fracture severity. MVCs and gunshot wounds contribute to a higher portion of severe facial fractures, whereas falls and sports-related accidents tend to be less severe. **Table 2** highlights the incidence of certain facial bone fractures. In this article, we focus on frontal, orbital, nasal, maxillofacial, and mandibular fractures.

FRONTAL BONE FRACTURES

Although the frontal bone is key to the facial architecture and aids in the transition between the facial skeleton and the cranium, it primarily serves as a part of the encasement for the brain and is part of the neurocranial bones. Fractures of the frontal bone are relatively infrequent, with various studies citing that they represent 5% to 15% of all facial fractures.[5,6] This is likely due to the anterior wall of the frontal sinus being capable of withstanding 800 to 2200 pounds of force, making it the strongest bone in the adult face.[6,7] Therefore, mechanisms of injury tend to involve high-velocity trauma, such as MVCs, assaults, and substantial falls. Several studies have shown that most frontal bone fractures (>90%) occur in men because they are more

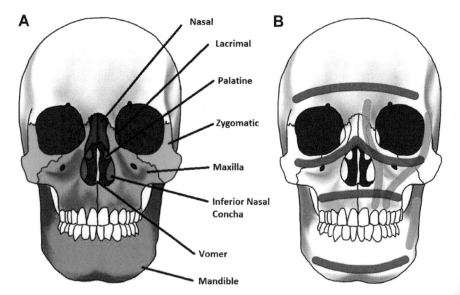

Fig. 1. Facial bone anatomy with horizontal and vertical buttresses. (*A*) The 14 bones that comprise the face. (*B*) The horizontal buttresses are in red; the left-sided vertical buttresses are in blue.

Table 1	
Factors influencing facial bone fracture epidemiology	
Protective Factors	**Risk Factors**
Vehicle restraint systems	Substance abuse
Airbags	Urban violence
Helmets	Increased all-terrain vehicle use
Sports protective equipment	International conflicts
Workplace safety regulations	

prone to be involved in car crashes, interpersonal violence, alcoholism, and drug abuse.[5,6,8]

Clinical Presentation

Patients presenting with an injury to the frontal bone often have obvious historical or physical examination elements that raise the clinician's suspicion for such a fracture. Most importantly, patients with trauma to the cranium should undergo a rapid assessment of their mental status. One small study reported that only 24% of patients with frontal bone fractures were conscious during their initial clinical evaluation.[9] Therefore, in patients with high-risk head trauma and altered mental status, there should be a low threshold to evaluate for concomitant intracranial and cervical spine pathology, as well as other traumatic injuries.

In awake patients with a frontal bone fracture, tenderness to palpation and edema over the frontal bone are the most common abnormalities (**Fig. 2**). Additionally, patients should be evaluated for cerebrospinal fluid (CSF) rhinorrhea. Damage to the cribriform plate may manifest as a postnasal drip or the taste of something sweet in the mouth. To evaluate nasal drainage for CSF, a halo test can be performed by placing a sample of the nasal fluid on filter paper or even a white sheet. If the fluid separates leaving a bloody center encircled by a "halo" of clear fluid there should be concern for a CSF leak (**Fig. 3**). Further confirmation includes testing the fluid for

Table 2							
Incidence of all-cause facial bone fractures							
	MVC	**Assault**	**Fall**	**Sports**	**Occupational**	**GSW**	**Total**
n =	319	365	129	62	26	28	929
Percentage of above							
Orbital	24.8	24.1	27.1	25.8	26.9	14.3	24.7
Mandibular	25.1	20.3	18.6	11.3	3.8	42.9	21.3
Nasal	13.8	15.1	29.5	38.7	11.5	0.0	17.7
Maxillary	13.5	19.5	7.8	9.7	19.2	28.6	15.4
Zygomaticomaxillary complex	8.8	7.7	8.5	8.1	11.5	3.6	8.2
Nasoethmoid orbital	6.0	5.2	2.3	1.6	11.5	3.6	5.0
Zygomatic arch	6.3	2.7	1.6	3.2	3.8	3.6	3.9
Frontal sinus	1.6	4.1	3.9	1.6	7.7	3.6	3.1
Other	0.3	1.4	0.8	0.0	3.8	0.0	0.9

Abbreviations: GSW, gunshot wound; MVC, motor vehicle collision.
From Erdmann D, Follmar KE, Debruijn M, et al. A retrospective analysis of facial fracture etiologies. Ann Plast Surg 2008;60(4):401; with permission.

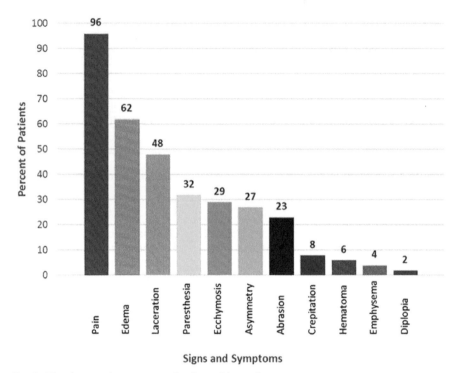

Fig. 2. The signs and symptoms of a frontal bone fracture.

glucose or β-2 transferrin.[10] Any of these findings should warrant prompt diagnostic imaging and a referral to neurosurgery, as a delay in the diagnosis of a frontal bone fracture can lead to sinusitis, hematoma, wound infection, persistent CSF leaks, and meningitis.[7]

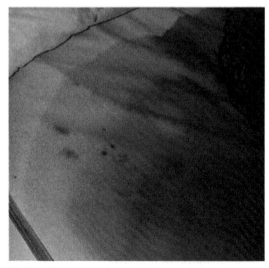

Fig. 3. A patient with head trauma and a positive halo test.

Imaging

A computed tomography (CT) scan is the gold standard in diagnosing a frontal bone fracture.[6] Given that fractures have a high association with other injuries, a CT scan of the brain, face, and/or cervical spine may be advised. Plain radiographs lack the ability to characterize the extent of fractures, detect nasofrontal involvement, and identify intracranial pathology.[11] One study showed that 3% of plain films negative for a skull fracture had fractures identified on CT. Of those, 50% went on to develop epidural hematomas, half of which required an operative intervention.[12] Finally, when clinical concern exists, CSF leaks may be identified by a CT myelogram.[6]

Initial Management

The ABCs of patient stabilization remain of paramount importance in a patient with suspected intracranial injuries. The treating clinician should be mindful of both advanced cardiac life support and advanced trauma life support protocols.

Consultation and Follow-up

Outside of individuals with altered mental status or intracranial involvement that warrant emergent neurosurgical evaluation, patients with identified frontal bone fractures (specifically those of the frontal sinus) require follow-up with a facial reconstructive surgeon. More than 58% of patients with frontal sinus fractures will require a surgical intervention.[11] The most common indications for surgery are a persistent CSF leak and a nasofrontal outflow tract injury with associated obstruction[6,9,11]

ORBITAL FRACTURES

Fractures involving the orbital bones are among the most common, if not the most common, injuries in facial trauma.[3,8,13] The orbit consists of 7 bones: frontal, sphenoid, maxilla, palatine, zygomatic, ethmoid, and lacrimal. Although fractures of any of these bones can occur, "blow-out" fractures are the most common type of orbital fractures (Fig. 4). They involve the weakest bones of the orbital wall, specifically the inferior and medial bones, and the lamina papyracea.[14] Less frequently, fracture fragments from the frontal or maxillary bones can cause a "blow-in" fracture.[15]

Clinical Presentation

An estimated 14% to 40% of blow-out fractures are associated with an ocular injury, and importantly, 5% to 10% of them result in a ruptured globe.[16,17] Therefore, the

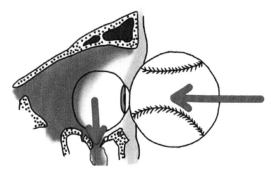

ig. 4. The forces of a blow-out fracture. The anterior to posterior force of the projectile roduces an inferior-directed force on the eye resulting in a blow-out fracture (Red arrows).

most important examination following ocular trauma entails an assessment of visual acuity. Reported injuries can include a ruptured globe, retrobulbar hematoma, hyphema, anterior chamber angle recession, lens dislocation, secondary glaucoma, vitreous hemorrhage, choroidal/retinal tear or detachment, and commotio retinae.[16] Thus, patients with reduced visual acuity should be emergently evaluated by an ophthalmologist.

The provider should next evaluate for areas of bony tenderness, swelling, and ecchymosis. Some patients with blow-out fractures may exhibit enophthalmos, which appears as depression of the globe secondary to sinking of the intraorbital fat through the orbital wall. Periorbital emphysema suggests fracture communication with the maxillary or ethmoid sinus. Additionally, patients should be checked for extraocular motion impairment, subconjunctival hemorrhage, and inferior orbital nerve paresthesia. Limitations of ocular movement or diplopia suggests ocular muscle entrapment.[18] The physical examination is critical when assessing for entrapment, as it is a clinical diagnosis.

Imaging

If an orbital fracture is suspected, patients should undergo a CT scan of the orbits with thin-sliced (1.5-mm) helical cuts.[19] Also, it is important for the clinician to consider whether other CT imaging of the face, head, and/or cervical spine is warranted to assess for concomitant injuries.

Initial Management

Any patient with concern for a ruptured globe, visual changes, and/or impaired ocular motion should be evaluated immediately by an ophthalmologist. Otherwise, individuals should be advised to sneeze with their mouths open, avoid nose blowing, and refrain from coughing or Valsalva maneuvers. Patients may apply ice to the affected area for 48 hours, use nasal decongestants, and use analgesics (eg, acetaminophen and ibuprofen while avoiding salicylic acid) to facilitate adequate pain control.[20] The use of prophylactic antibiotics is still debated, but a 5-day course of cephalexin or amoxicillin-clavulanate is commonly prescribed.[21,22]

Consultation and Follow-up

If ocular injury has been ruled out and imaging confirms an orbital fracture, patients should follow-up with ophthalmology or maxillofacial surgery within 1 week.[18] This allows for the patient's swelling to resolve, facilitating a better assessment of the remaining symptoms. Approximately 50% of patients experience resolution of their symptoms and are managed non-operatively; however, persistent diplopia on primary gaze at 2 weeks postinjury is managed operatively.[23]

In children younger than 7 years, the orbital bones tend to be more malleable. Although this flexibility reduces the likelihood of an orbital fracture, it does increase the incidence of extraocular muscle entrapment. Providers should have a high index of suspicion for entrapment in children with diplopia or activation of the oculocardiac reflex (ie, bradycardia in response to traction from entrapment of the ocular muscles).[24] Orbital fractures can lead to permanent extraocular motion limitation, diplopia, orbital infection, and/or cosmetic defects such as an enophthalmos.[25] Approximately 15% of these patients will require a surgical intervention, and a delay in diagnosis or failure to secure follow-up can lead to permanent visual changes.

NASAL BONE FRACTURES

The nose is the most prominent aesthetic feature of the face and is quite susceptible to injury. The nasal bone is the most commonly fractured facial bone, and the third most commonly fractured bone in the human body.[3,8,10,18,26] Composed of very thin bone, nasal fractures happen frequently and with minimal force.

Nasal bone fractures commonly occur from blunt trauma. Young males are more likely to sustain a nasal injury with the peak incidence occurring in the 20s to 30s.[8,10,13] Some of the increased prevalence of nasal fractures stems from increasing participation in competitive and high-velocity sports in this demographic.[27]

A specific classification system for nasal bone fracture does not exist.[28] It is best to define the degree and severity of injury by the number and complexity of the identified fractures, degree of displacement, and concomitant injuries (including possible lacerations). Low-velocity injuries (eg, elbow to the nose) may lead to a simple fracture pattern. High-velocity injuries tend to be associated with more complex fractures. It is important to evaluate for a concomitant airway obstruction, CSF rhinorrhea, or a septal hematoma, especially in more severe nasal injuries.[10]

Clinical Presentation

Within the first few hours (before the onset of significant edema), it is possible for the clinician to fully evaluate the site of injury and perform a closed reduction, if necessary; however, once edema has set in, swelling can distort the shape of the nose. In those instances, most interventions should be deferred until the edema resolves.[10] Individuals with nasal bone fractures may also have some degree of nasal airway obstruction. Secondary signs suggestive of a nasal fracture include epistaxis, a visible or palpable deformity, and tenderness to palpation of the nose.

It is important for the clinician to inspect the nose for both external and internal abnormalities. Externally, the clinician should look for any deformities, displacement, and lacerations. Palpation of the nose for step-offs, crepitus, and tenderness are the most certain signs of fracture. Internally, both nasal passageways should be evaluated for epistaxis, septal hematoma, and CSF rhinorrhea. It is imperative to promptly drain septal hematomas because a failure to do so could result in septal cartilage avascular necrosis (Refer to chapter 11). Any significant clear drainage from the nose should increase one's suspicion for CSF rhinorrhea. This may be further confirmed via the halo test (see **Fig. 3**) and/or testing the fluid for glucose or β-2 transferrin.

Imaging

In general, imaging is not necessary to diagnose an isolated nasal bone fracture. An emergency medicine study reported that plain radiographs do not significantly change the diagnosis or management of nasal fratures.[29] High-resolution ultrasonography (**Fig. 5**) has been shown to possess an accuracy rate of 100% for nasal fractures compared with 92% in CT.[30] Patients with complex nasal injuries and/or other associated facial fractures should undergo a maxillofacial CT scan to fully characterize the extent of any additional injuries.

Initial Management

The initial management of nasal fractures entails first treating a septal hematoma or epistaxis, if present. Once those sequelae are addressed, a closed-fracture reduction can be entertained. The goals of this procedure include an acceptable cosmetic appearance, bilateral nasal airway patency, and prevention of intranasal

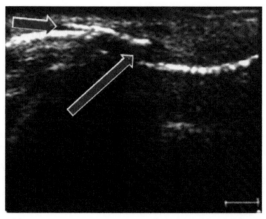

Fig. 5. Ultrasound imaging of the nose revealing 2 fractures (*purple arrows*).

stenosis or septal perforation.[31] Attempting reduction within the first few hours is ideal; however, once edema has set in, a closed reduction should be deferred. In such circumstances, a provider should recommend analgesic medications, prescribe antibiotics for any open wounds (eg, cephalexin), provide instructions regarding the use of ice and head elevation, and facilitate follow-up in 5 to 7 days with an otolaryngologist.[32]

If a closed-fracture reduction is attempted, it is important to counsel the patient appropriately. Patients will likely experience pain and discomfort and should be advised that the procedure can be deferred until follow-up in 5 to 7 days.[27] Attempts at a reduction can worsen epistaxis and, even if a reduction is attempted, 14% to 50% of patients may require rhinoplasty or septorhinoplasty.[33] Other research, however, found 79% to 91% of patients were satisfied with the outcome of a closed-fracture reduction attempt in the ED, and only 3% proceeded to surgical intervention at 3 years.[34,35]

Before a closed reduction, it is imperative to provide adequate anesthesia. Several options exist: topical cocaine, 1% lidocaine with epinephrine, a hematoma block with 1% lidocaine with epinephrine, and bilateral infraorbital nerve blocks[27] (**Fig. 6**). The provider then places the palmar surface of the thumb against the lateralized segment of the nasal bone as the remaining fingers extend over the contralateral zygomatic process (**Fig. 7**). Then, broad and gentle pressure is exerted at the bony step-off until the nasal bone appears symmetric or returns to the desired position. An audible or palpable click may be appreciated. This reduction approach may fail if the fractured fragments overlap or the reduction requires lateralization of a fracture fragment.[27]

Consultation and Follow-up

Patients should be advised to keep their head and nose elevated to help minimize edema. Ice will both reduce edema and provide analgesia. Nasal decongestants should be recommended. Some advocate for broad-spectrum antibiotics (eg, cephalexin, amoxicillin-clavulanate, or clindamycin) for 7 days, especially in the setting of an open fracture.[10,32]

Patients who may warrant urgent evaluation by an otolaryngologist include those with a delayed presentation, evidence of comminuted facial fractures, an untreated septal hematoma and/or abscess, persistent epistaxis, nasal obstruction, and a CSF leak.[27]

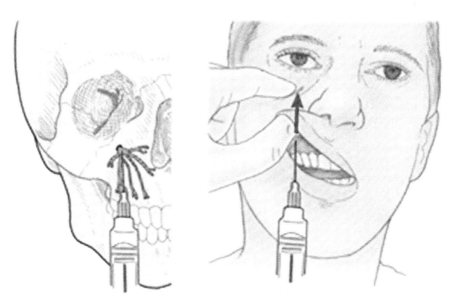

Fig. 6. External (*left*) and intraoral (*right*) infraorbital nerve block entry locations.

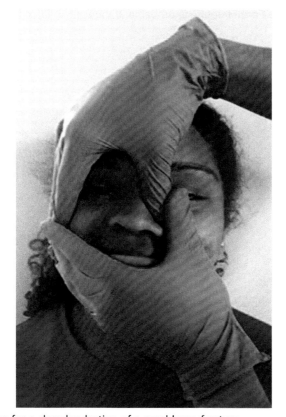

Fig. 7. Technique for a closed reduction of a nasal bone fracture.

MAXILLOFACIAL FRACTURES

The maxillofacial region includes most of the bones in the face (see **Fig. 1**), excluding the mandible. This area, termed the midface, is encircled by the frontal bone, the paired zygoma, and the maxillary bones.[2] This section discusses fractures involving the maxilla and zygoma.

It is estimated that 30% of facial fractures involve the midface.[15] These injuries are more commonly seen in younger male individuals, with fractures of the zygoma being among the most common, second only to mandibular fractures.[2–4,8,13,36] Many midface fractures are complex and are more likely to have concomitant injuries.[2,13,37] To help classify these potentially complex fractures, the Le Fort system was developed to describe midface fractures involving the maxilla[2] (**Fig. 8**).

Clinical Presentation

Clinical features of maxillary and zygomatic fractures are listed in **Table 3**. Because the maxilla supports the pharyngeal constrictor and palatal muscles, its posterior and inferior displacement can result in airway compromise. Zygomatic fractures can affect the extraocular muscles and thus a patient's vision. Importantly, although CSF rhinorrhea is rare, it may accompany maxillofacial fractures.

To evaluate for a Le Fort fracture, the clinician should place one hand on the patient's nasal bridge and use the other to manipulate the maxillary teeth. If only the maxilla moves, the patient likely has a Le Fort I fracture. If both the nasal bridge and maxilla move, a Le Fort II fracture is probable. If the entire midface moves (including

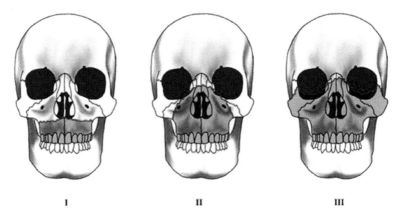

I   II   III

Le Fort Fracture Definitions

Type	Description
I (Horizontal)	Fracture of the maxilla below the nose and above the teeth
	Fracture extends through the lateral maxillary sinus to the lateral pterygoid plate
II (Pyramidal)	Pyramid-shaped fracture from the nasal and ethmoid bones
	Additional fracture through the zygomaticomaxillary suture and maxilla
III (Transverse)	Craniofacial disjunction causing movement of the entire midface
	Fracture extends horizontally through the orbital rims and the base of the nose

Fig. 8. The Le Fort fracture classifications.

Table 3
The signs and symptoms of a midface fracture

Signs of a Maxillary Fracture	Signs of a Zygomatic Fracture
Pain with jaw motion	Pain over the cheekbone
Bleeding from oral or gingival mucosa	Depression of the cheekbone or step-off of the infraorbital rim
Epistaxis	Periorbital and maxillary vestibular ecchymosis or edema
Loose, fractured, or displaced teeth	Diplopia, orbital dystopia, enophthalmos, or proptosis
Inability to chew or malocclusion	Extraocular muscle movement abnormalities
Facial elongation with maxilla displacement posteroinferiorly	Subconjunctival hemorrhage
Infraorbital nerve paresthesia	Infraorbital nerve paresthesia

the orbital rims) a Le Fort III fracture should be suspected.[38] Individuals may possess different Le Fort fractures on each side of the face at the same time.

Imaging

The gold standard for identifying maxillofacial fractures is a maxillofacial CT with 2-mm axial and coronal cuts.[2,38] Also, given the high association of intraorbital pathology with zygomatic fractures, detailed orbital CT imaging should be considered.[39]

Initial Management

Injuries resulting in significant bleeding should be controlled with gentle pressure and elevation of the head, protecting the cervical spine when necessary. Care should be taken to avoid shifting or worsening any fracture positioning.

Consultation and Follow-up

Nearly all midface fractures require prompt consultation with an oral maxillofacial surgeon. The exceptions are closed zygoma fractures, even if displaced, which are considered stable for outpatient reduction in 1 to 3 days. Because more than 90% of patients with midface fractures sustain ocular injuries of varying severity, consultation with an ophthalmologist should be strongly entertained. Midface fractures are typically managed with open reduction and internal fixation.[39]

MANDIBULAR FRACTURES

Mandibular fractures are the second most common injury in facial trauma. However, they are the most common fracture site in assault and gunshot injuries.[3,36] Young males are disproportionally affected, with the highest incidence involving 16 and 30-year olds.[8,13,15]

The frequency of the precise anatomic site of the mandibular fracture varies among sources. It is generally agreed that 75% to 90% of fractures occur in a relatively even distribution between the mandibular condyle, body, and angle[2,40] (**Fig. 9**). The mandible is a ringlike structure, and thus it is important to suspect contralateral fractures. Overall, an estimated 20% to 40% of patients with mandibular fractures have additional injuries. Intracranial injuries (39%), lacerations (30%), midface fractures (28%), ocular injuries (16%), nasal fractures (12%), and cervical spine fractures (11%) have been shown to be relatively common in this context.[40]

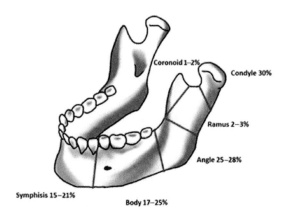

Fig. 9. Distribution of mandibular fractures.

Clinical Presentation

Individuals with mandibular fractures may report pain exacerbated by jaw movement, dysphagia, and/or an abnormal alignment of their bite. It is important to inspect the jaw for asymmetry, crepitus, step-offs, and lacerations. **Box 1** lists physical examination findings associated with mandibular fractures.

The tongue blade bite test can be used to rule out mandible fractures given its excellent sensitivity. The test is performed by inserting a tongue depressor between the maxillary and mandibular teeth, then asking the patient to bite down. The clinician then twists the blade, and if the tongue depressor can be cracked without eliciting pain, the test is considered negative for a fracture. Several studies have shown the test to have a sensitivity of 88% to 95% and a negative predictive value of 92% to 100%.[41,42]

Imaging

An orthopantomogram (ie, Panorex) can help facilitate both the diagnosis and surgical planning of a mandibular fracture, possessing a sensitivity of 92%.[2,43] When there is

---

Box 1
The signs and symptoms of a mandibular fracture

Trismus

Bleeding from lacerated gingival or mucosal tissue

Ecchymosis/hematoma (at the fracture site or the sublingual space)

Loose, fractured, or displaced teeth

Palpable or visible "step" in the dental arch

Inability to chew or subjective (or obvious) altered bite

Paresthesia of the lip/chin

Lack of motion of the mandibular condyles with palpation through the external auditory canal

From Viozzi CF. Maxillofacial and mandibular fractures in sports. Clin Sports Med 2017;36(2):355–68.

high clinical suspicion for a fracture in the setting of a negative orthopantomogram, a maxillofacial CT should be obtained. This is secondary to reports of more identified fractures on CT when there is no fracture identified on orthopantomogram (96% vs 81%).[44] The clinical utility of the CT scan is particularly evident when evaluating for ramus or condyle fractures, as the degree of displacement in these areas can be subtle.[2] Of note, if the patient undergoes a CT to evaluate for blunt head injury and/or cervical spine pathology, the addition of a maxillofacial CT may be the most logical and simple approach.

Initial Management

Oral bleeding should be addressed by having the patient bite on gauze. If a dental disruption is suspected with a mandibular fracture, alveolar ridge fracture, or a laceration, these are considered to be open fractures. Accordingly, initial wound closure should be delayed. Antibiotics to cover oral microbes should be given (eg, clindamycin), and the patient may even warrant intravenous antibiotics (eg, ampicillin/sulbactam). Keeping the individual's mouth closed may decrease the risk for further fracture displacement. With these initial steps, the clinician is attempting to prevent many of the sequelae of mandibular fractures, including infection, disruption of dental roots, dental abscess, pulp necrosis, malocclusion, malunion, and nonunion.[15]

Consultation and Follow-up

Nearly all patients with mandibular fractures should be emergently evaluated by an otolaryngologist or an oral maxillofacial surgeon. Although the definitive management for mandibular fractures ranges from nonoperative observation with soft dietary and functional restrictions to internal or external fixation, more than 90% of patients are managed operatively. The most common approach for a surgical repair is intraoral fixation.[45] Infrequently, patients with nondisplaced, closed fractures and minimal pain can be discharged from the ED to follow-up with otolaryngology or oral maxillofacial surgery.

SUMMARY

Facial trauma is not a rare occurrence in the ED, and it carries significant risk to patients both with regard to facial fractures and injuries involving the brain, cervical spine, eyes, and other nearby anatomic structures The clinician must first evaluate the ABCs, stabilize the cervical spine when necessary, control significant bleeding, and then proceed to assess for facial fractures. Frontal, orbital, nasal, maxillofacial, and mandibular fractures each possess unique aspects to their evaluation and management. When assessing these injuries, providers should keenly observe for palpable defects, ecchymosis, edema, evidence of an open fracture, and the presence of CSF. A CT scan is often the diagnostic modality of choice, although there are occasional instances when plain film radiography can be valuable (eg, mandibular fractures). When the diagnosis is confirmed, facial fractures are frequently accompanied by the need to consult an otolaryngologist, oral maxillofacial surgeon, and/or an ophthalmologist. The timely and appropriate utilization of these consultants can help to minimize a patient's risk of long-term morbidity and mortality.

REFERENCES

1. Allareddy V, Allareddy V, Nalliah RP. Epidemiology of facial fracture injuries. J Oral Maxillofac Surg 2011;69(10):2613–8.

2. Viozzi CF. Maxillofacial and mandibular fractures in sports. Clin Sports Med 2017; 36(2):355–68.
3. Erdmann D, Follmar KE, Debruijn M, et al. A retrospective analysis of facial fracture etiologies. Ann Plast Surg 2008;60(4):398–403.
4. Murphy C, O'Connell JE, Kearns G, et al. Sports-related maxillofacial injuries. J Craniofac Surg 2015;26(7):2120–3.
5. Marinheiro BH, de Medeiros EH, Sverzut CE, et al. Frontal bone fractures. J Craniofac Surg 2014;25(6):2139–43.
6. Schultz K, Braun TL, Truong TA. Frontal sinus fractures. Semin Plast Surg 2017; 31(2):80–4.
7. Guy WM, Brissett AE. Contemporary management of traumatic fractures of the frontal sinus. Otolaryngol Clin North Am 2013;46(5):733–48.
8. Montovani JC, de Campos LM, Gomes MA, et al. Etiology and incidence facial fractures in children and adults. Braz J Otorhinolaryngol 2006;72(2):235–41.
9. Rohrich RJ, Hollier LH. Management of frontal sinus fractures. Changing concepts. Clin Plast Surg 1992;19(1):219–32.
10. Higuera S, Lee EI, Cole P, et al. Nasal trauma and the deviated nose. Plast Reconstr Surg 2007;120(7 Suppl 2):64s–75s.
11. Rodriguez ED, Stanwix MG, Nam AJ, et al. Twenty-six-year experience treating frontal sinus fractures: a novel algorithm based on anatomical fracture pattern and failure of conventional techniques. Plast Reconstr Surg 2008;122(6): 1850–66.
12. Nakahara K, Shimizu S, Utsuki S, et al. Linear fractures occult on skull radiographs: a pitfall at radiological screening for mild head injury. J Trauma 2011; 70(1):180–2.
13. Brook IM, Wood N. Aetiology and incidence of facial fractures in adults. Int J Oral Surg 1983;12(5):293–8.
14. Nikolaenko VP, Astakhov YS. Orbital fractures: a physician's manual. Berlin: Springer Berlin Heidelberg; 2015.
15. Bracker MD. 5-minute sports medicine consult. Philadelphia: Wolters Kluwer Health; 2015.
16. Brady SM, McMann MA, Mazzoli RA, et al. The diagnosis and management of orbital blowout fractures: update 2001. Am J Emerg Med 2001;19(2):147–54.
17. Rosen P, Barkin RM, Schaider J. Rosen & Barkin's 5-minute emergency medicine consult, 3rd edition. Philadelphia: Wolters Kluwer Health; 2007.
18. Louis M, Agrawal N, Kaufman M, et al. Midface fractures I. Semin Plast Surg 2017;31(2):85–93.
19. Go JL, Vu VN, Lee KJ, et al. Orbital trauma. Neuroimaging Clin N Am 2002;12(2): 311–24.
20. Jatla KK, Enzenauer RW. Orbital fractures: a review of current literature. Curr Surg 2004;61(1):25–9.
21. Mundinger GS, Borsuk DE, Okhah Z, et al. Antibiotics and facial fractures: evidence-based recommendations compared with experience-based practice. Craniomaxillofac Trauma Reconstr 2015;8(1):64–78.
22. Reiss B, Rajjoub L, Mansour T, et al. Antibiotic prophylaxis in orbital fractures. Open Ophthalmol J 2017;11:11–6.
23. Choi M, Flores RL. Medial orbital wall fractures and the transcaruncular approach. J Craniofac Surg 2012;23(3):696–701.
24. Feldmann ME, Rhodes JL. Pediatric orbital floor fracture. Eplasty 2012;12:ic9.
25. Linden JA, Renner GS. Trauma to the globe. Emerg Med Clin North Am 1995; 13(3):581–605.

26. Dingman RO, Grabb WC, Oneal RM. Management of injuries of the naso-orbital complex. Arch Surg 1969;98(5):566–71.
27. Marston AP, O'Brien EK, Hamilton GS 3rd. Nasal injuries in sports. Clin Sports Med 2017;36(2):337–53.
28. Murray JA, Maran AG, Busuttil A, et al. A pathological classification of nasal fractures. Injury 1986;17(5):338–44.
29. Logan M, O'Driscoll K, Masterson J. The utility of nasal bone radiographs in nasal trauma. Clin Radiol 1994;49(3):192–4.
30. Hee LM, Gyu CJ, Sook HH, et al. Comparison of high-resolution ultrasonography and computed tomography in the diagnosis of nasal fractures. J Ultrasound Med 2009;28(6):717–23.
31. Bailey BJ, Healy GB, Johnson JT, et al. Head and neck surgery - otolaryngology. Philadelphia: Lippincott Williams & Wilkins; 2001.
32. Stewart MG. Head, face, and neck trauma: comprehensive management. New York: Thieme; 2005.
33. Rohrich RJ, Adams WP Jr. Nasal fracture management: minimizing secondary nasal deformities. Plast Reconstr Surg 2000;106(2):266–73.
34. Illum P. Long-term results after treatment of nasal fractures. J Laryngol Otol 1986; 100(3):273–7.
35. Staffel JG. Optimizing treatment of nasal fractures. Laryngoscope 2002;112(10): 1709–19.
36. Lee K. Global trends in maxillofacial fractures. Craniomaxillofac Trauma Reconstr 2012;5(4):213–22.
37. Reehal P. Facial injury in sport. Curr Sports Med Rep 2010;9(1):27–34.
38. Louis M, Agrawal N, Truong TA. Midface fractures II. Semin Plast Surg 2017; 31(2):94–9.
39. al-Qurainy IA, Stassen LF, Dutton GN, et al. The characteristics of midfacial fractures and the association with ocular injury: a prospective study. Br J Oral Maxillofac Surg 1991;29(5):291–301.
40. Fridrich KL, Pena-Velasco G, Olson RA. Changing trends with mandibular fractures: a review of 1,067 cases. J Oral Maxillofac Surg 1992;50(6):586–9.
41. Neiner J, Free R, Caldito G, et al. Tongue blade bite test predicts mandible fractures. Craniomaxillofac Trauma Reconstr 2016;9(2):121–4.
42. Caputo ND, Raja A, Shields C, et al. Re-evaluating the diagnostic accuracy of the tongue blade test: still useful as a screening tool for mandibular fractures? J Emerg Med 2013;45(1):8–12.
43. Chayra GA, Meador LR, Laskin DM. Comparison of panoramic and standard radiographs for the diagnosis of mandibular fractures. J Oral Maxillofac Surg 1986; 44(9):677–9.
44. Roth FS, Kokoska MS, Awwad EE, et al. The identification of mandible fractures by helical computed tomography and panorex tomography. J Craniofac Surg 2005;16(3):394–9.
45. Munante-Cardenas JL, Facchina Nunes PH, Passeri LA. Etiology, treatment, and complications of mandibular fractures. J Craniofac Surg 2015;26(3):611–5.

Printed and bound by CPI Group (UK) Ltd, Croydon, CR0 4YY

08/05/2025

01864737-0002